Acupuncture: Treatment of Musculoskeletal Conditions

Acquisitions editor: Heidi Allen
Development editor: Myriam Brearley
Production controller: Anthony Read
Desk editor: Jane Campbell
Cover designer: Helen Brockway

Acupuncture: Treatment of Musculoskeletal Conditions

Christopher M. Norris
MSC, CAc, MCSP, SRP

Director of Norris Associates, Chartered Physiotherapists,
Sale, Cheshire, UK

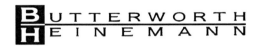

OXFORD AUCKLAND BOSTON JOHANNESBURG MELBOURNE NEW DELHI

Butterworth-Heinemann
Linacre House, Jordan Hill, Oxford OX2 8DP
225 Wildwood Avenue, Woburn, MA 01801-2041

 A division of Reed Educational and Professional Publishing Ltd

First published 2001

Reed Educational and Professional Publishing Ltd 2001

British Library Cataloguing in Publication Data
Norris, Christopher M.
    Acupuncture: treatment of musculoskeletal conditions
    1. Acupuncture   2.   Musculoskeletal system – Acupuncture
    I.Title
    615.8′92

Library of Congress Cataloguing in Publication Data
Norris, Christopher M.
    Acupuncture: treatment of musculoskeletal conditions/Christopher M. Norris.
    p.; cm.
    Includes bibliographical references and index.
    ISBN 0 7506 5173 3
    1. Acupuncture.   2.   Physical therapy.   3.   Musculoskeletal system – Diseases – Treatment.
    I. Title
    [DNLM 1.   Acupuncture Points.   2.   Acupuncture Therapy – methods.   3.   Musculoskeletal
    Diseases – therapy.   WB 369 N854a 2001]
    RM184. N8956
    615.8′92–dc21

                                                                                                    2001035735

ISBN 0 7506 5173 3

Transferred to digital printing in 2006.

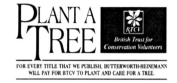

Contents

Introduction

This book is written primarily for musculoskeletal therapists of all types, and will appeal to those who use acupuncture to augment their current practice. It will also be of value to acupuncturists specialising in the treatment of musculoskeletal conditions, and may serve as an introduction to physical treatment methods such as joint mobilisation, therapeutic exercise and taping.

I have deliberately placed acupuncture and physical therapy procedures side by side in Chapters 8, 9 and 10, to allow practitioners to bring acupuncture treatment alongside their current practice. It is my firm belief that acupuncture greatly increases the effectiveness of physical therapy, but cannot replace it. To combine acupuncture with physical therapy gives a far better clinical outcome than to use either technique in isolation.

In this book I have tried to achieve a balance between Traditional Chinese Acupuncture and Western Medical Acupuncture. Physiotherapists in particular often limit their acupuncture to western needling methods treating trigger points and local painful areas. Although effective, this approach often fails to achieve a long-term result. By appreciating the basic principles of Traditional Chinese medicine (TCM), acupuncture can be extended to give even greater effects. In addition, by applying TCM principles, linked symptoms are often revealed which show a musculoskeletal pain as part of a larger holistic picture of disorder. In many cases this can allow the practitioner to identify and treat conditions which could not previously be helped by physical therapy.

Chapters 1 and 2 give the basics of TCM which can form a foundation for further study. The description of meridian channels in Chapter 3 and acupuncture points in Chapter 5 take a western anatomical approach. Accurate palpation skills are assumed, and those practitioners who do not possess these will find that they need to learn or revise surface anatomy to be able to localise points with precision. Chapter 5 looks at pain from both a traditional Chinese and western medical approach, and highlights the similarities and differences between the two systems. Chapter 6 looks at patient questioning and point selection and is intended to act as an extension to the subjective examination that therapists already use in their day to day practice. Chapter 7, describing acupuncture treatment methods should act as an introduction and by no means covers all available techniques.

The treatment protocols described in Chapters 8, 9 and 10 are designed to guide the practitioner without being a simplistic 'cookbook'. As such, treatment suggestions must be modified depending on the results of subjective and objective examination. In addition as treatment progresses, point selection may change as the patient's condition changes.

In writing this book it is my aim firstly to encourage the combined use of acupuncture and physical therapy in the treatment of musculoskeletal conditions. Secondly, by encouraging the 'dual use' I hope to spur an improvement in the standard of clinical practice by both physical and acupuncture therapists. If these aims can be achieved, the patient will be the ultimate beneficiary.

List of abbreviations

A/C	Acromioclavicular joint
ASIS	Anterior superior iliac spine
CMC	Carpo-metacarpal joint
CSF	Cerebrospinal fluid
CT	Computerised tomography
EA	Electroacupuncture
EDL	Extensor digitorum longus
EOP	External occipital protuberance
5-HT	5-Hydroxytryptamine (serotonin)
ITB	Ilio-tibial band
LBP	Low back pain
MCL	Medial collateral ligament
MP	Metatarsal phalangeal joint
PIIS	Posterior inferior iliac spine
PSIS	Posterior superior iliac spine
S/C	Sternoclavicular joint
SG	Substantia gelaninosa
SIJ	Sacro-iliac joint
STJ	Subtaloid joint
TCM	Traditional Chinese medicine
TENS	Transcutaneous electrical nerve stimulation
TMJ	Temporo-mandibular joint
TrP	Trigger point
VMO	Vastus medialis obliqus
WDR	Wide dynamic range

Principles of traditional Chinese medicine

Introduction

In order to understand the methods used in acupuncture it is helpful to have a basic understanding of traditional Chinese medicine (TCM) as it is within this scheme that acupuncture has its roots. Although this book does not pretend to be a reference work on the many faces of TCM, the following chapter will attempt to give some insights into the fundamental features of this fascinating system of healing.

Vital substances

Qi

Variously translated as 'vital energy' or 'vital substance', qi is central to all aspects of TCM. Qi is both substance (solid) and non-substance (spirit or energy) at the same time. Although seemingly alien to western medical thinking, this concept is not so far removed from modern descriptions of the universe in quantum physics. In both situations the universe is seen to exist on a continuum from pure energy at one end through to solid matter at the other. The ancient Chinese saw the universe as a continual coming together (aggregation) and moving apart (dispersion) of qi, resulting in varying states of matter and energy. The important fact in both TCM and quantum physics models is that matter and energy are continuous and not separate items. This being the case, the possibility exists that one can change into the other, and this fact has been highlighted in the west by Einstein's theory of relativity. Many people will recognise the equation $E = MC^2$ without necessarily knowing its meaning. Put simply, this equation is a demonstration of the very real direct relationship between matter and energy.

The ancient Chinese saw this relationship as central to life and to TCM, and a number of Chinese philosophers have described and discussed this relationship in considerable detail. In 1000AD Zhang Zai (quoted in Maciocia, 1989) wrote that the universe consisted of qi where '*qi condenses to become the myriad things. Things . . . disintegrate and return to the great void.*' Human life was seen as no different to this '*every birth is a condensation, every death a dispersal. Birth is not a gain, death is not a loss.*'

This continuity of solid to energy is important to TCM. If qi circulation is poor, qi will condense and come together to form a mass either less dense (muscle nodule) or more dense (tumour) depending on the severity and type of stagnation. The solid aspect of qi in the body is produced by the internal organs to nourish the body while the energy aspect of qi is the functional activity of the organs themselves. There are thus several types of qi relevant to the location and function of the qi at any one time. Each organ has a qi attributed to it, thus there is 'liver qi' and 'heart qi' meaning the function of these organs (see Chapter 2). There are also several named types of qi which are specific to different regions of the body.

Classification of qi

Qi may be either congenital or acquired. Congenital qi, also known as *primary qi* or 'yuan qi' is derived from our parents. Primary qi stimulates and promotes the activity of the Zang Fu organs, while the organs themselves nourish the primary qi, the relationship being one of interdependence. Primary qi is stored in the kidney and spreads through the body via the triple energizer (sanjiao) meridian. From here it is passed to the meridians and stored in the source points (yuan points) of each meridian. An abundance of primary qi will give vibrant good health, while on the other hand depletion of primary qi (through congenital insufficiency or prolonged ill health) will lead to pathology of various types.

Three types of acquired qi are generally described. Pectoral or *Chest qi* (Zong qi) is formed by combining clean qi obtained through inspiration by the lung with qi from food transformed by the spleen. Chest qi is stored in the chest region and functions to promote the activity of the lungs and heart described in Chapter 2. *Nutrient qi* (ying qi) is obtained from the food, it is the refined 'essence' of food and water. The stomach separates the nutrient qi from food and passes it to the spleen for transportation around the body. The primary function of nutrient qi is to produce blood and to circulate with it. Finally, *defensive qi* (Wei qi, or 'anti-pathogenic' qi) is also derived from the food, but unlike nutrient qi it does not circulate in the blood vessels, but outside them. It works to protect the body surface (muscles and skin) against the invasion of external pathogenic factors (see Chapter 4). Defensive qi controls the opening and closing of the pores of the skin and also moistens the skin and hair. Defensive qi does not flow in the meridians, but between the skin and muscle, hence its effect on sweating. Defensive qi and nutrient qi are intimately related. They both come from the same source, but defensive qi circulates outside the meridian system and guards the *exterior* (it is therefore said to 'belong to *yang*') while nutrient qi circulates within the meridian system providing nutrient for the *interior* and belongs to *yin* (see page 6).

Movement of qi is in four directions, and changes in these movements can cause or be part of pathology in TCM. The four directions of qi movement are upward (ascending), downward (descending), exiting (outward), and entering (inward). Each organ contributes to this movement in total or in part. For example the stomach qi descends while spleen qi ascends. Disharmony of qi will result in changes to the normal direction of qi flow (counterflow qi). If qi ascends too much this is called 'abnormal qi rising' while over-descending is called 'sinking qi'. Too much outward movement is 'escape of qi' while too much inward movement is 'qi accumulation'. Lack of qi movement is known as 'qi stagnation' and is a common cause of pain in TCM (see Chapter 4).

The zang fu organs themselves have their own qi, formed from congenital and acquired qi. It is the organ qi which circulates in the meridian system. The organ qi is formed from food essence, inhaled qi and essential qi stored in the kidney. The organ qi is referred to as 'vital qi' (Zheng qi) and is the basis of meridian acupuncture treatment.

Table 1.1. Functions of qi.

Promoting	Promotes and stimulates growth and development in general and all physiological functions.
Warming	Qi warms the whole body. If qi is deficient the patient will show an aversion to cold and cold sensations in the limbs.
Defending	Defends the body surface against pathogenic attack.
Checking	Controls and regulates body substances, such as sweat and urine. If qi is deficient, the patient may show spontaneous sweating and incontinence.
Nourishing	Qi nourishes the whole body. If qi is deficient the body is not nourished and chronic illness results.

Qi has five main general functions described in Table 1.1. Each of the four types of qi has specific functions as well. Primary qi activates growth and development and promotes the functional activities of the zang fu organs; its function is reflected by that of the kidney. It is the motivating power behind the vital activities of the body. Chest qi has effects centered on the lung and heart. It flows into the respiratory tract to promote respiration and to support the voice. In addition it flows into the heart to cause the heartbeat and blood circulation. Nutrient qi has two functions. One is to produce blood and it in itself becomes a component of blood and travels with it. The second function is to nourish the whole body. Defensive qi protects the body surface and combats pathogens. Examples of qi pathology are shown in Table 1.2.

Table 1.2. Pathology of qi.

Qi deficiency	Insufficient qi normally of spleen, lungs or kidneys.
Sinking qi	Failure to 'hold up' organs giving rise to prolapse.
Qi stagnation	Too little qi movement, normally due to liver qi.
Rebellious qi	Qi flowing in wrong direction. For example, stomach qi flowing upwards rather than downwards and causing nausea and vomiting.

Essence

Essence (jing) is the fundamental material of the human body, and includes congenital or 'pre-heaven' essence and essence refined from food and water, known as 'post heaven' essence. Congenital essence comes from the mother and father and fuses at conception. Only congenital essence is present in the foetus. From birth the child has access to acquired essence which is refined and extracted from food, water, and air. Acquired essence is closely related to the functions of the stomach and spleen in 'decomposing' food and 'transforming' it (see page 17). The two types of essence combine to form kidney essence, sometimes simply referred to as 'essence'. Essence is stored in the kidney and circulates freely throughout the body, and controls reproduction and development (sexual maturation).

It can be seen that qi and essence have many similarities, but a variety of differences exist. Essence is said to be fluid-like in consistency whereas qi is energy. Essence is therefore free to circulate by itself while qi requires blood as its vehicle. Essence resides mostly in the kidneys and travels from here, while qi is found throughout the body and in each Zang Fu organ. Qi moves and changes/reacts quickly whereas changes in essence occur much more slowly (Maciocia, 1989).

Blood

The function of blood in TCM is similar to that of western medicine, but the substance itself is different. Qi infuses into the blood and is carried by it, so that blood and qi are inseparable. Blood is made from the food by the stomach and spleen. The fluid nature of blood means that it is similar to essence, and may transform into essence in the kidney. Essence in turn may transform into blood in the liver. Blood circulation is dominated by the heart while the spleen controls the blood and prevents it leaking from the blood vessels (extravasation). The liver stores the blood and controls blood volume. Disorders of the liver, spleen or heart may affect the blood in a variety of ways. Deficiency of the heart qi may lead to blood stagnation while dysfunction of the spleen in controlling blood may lead to bruising or blood in the stools.

Table 1.3. Pathology of blood, and tongue diagnosis findings.

Blood deficiency	Not enough manufactured, normally due to spleen deficiency. Thin tongue body.
Blood heat	Due to liver heat. Red/purple tongue.
Blood stasis	Movement too slow. Due to stagnation of liver qi or due to heat or cold. Tongue purple.

Blood is said to nourish and moisten the body tissues, and be the foundation for mental activities. This is why deficiency of blood can give psychological effects in TCM. For example deficiency of heart or liver blood may give insomnia and mental restlessness. The inseparable nature of qi and blood is also illustrated clinically. After heavy exertion for example, which depletes qi, signs of blood deficiency are seen including pallor and dizziness. Similarly after massive blood loss, qi deficiency is seen demonstrated by sweating and cold limbs. Examples of blood pathology are shown in Table 1.3.

Body fluids

Body fluids (Jinye) in TCM consist of two parts. 'Jin' is dilute fluid which flows easily and has a *moistening* function; in western medicine this would be normal tissue fluid flowing into the lymph system. 'Ye' is thicker, more dense tissue fluid which flows less easily and has a *nourishing* function. In western medicine this would equate with joint (synovial) fluid, and cerebrospinal fluid (CSF). Body fluid helps with the regulation of body temperature through sweating and the excretion of waste products through the pores.

Body fluid is formed through a series of purification processes. It is the function of the stomach to form body fluid initially. As food is taken in, the 'pure' part is passed to the spleen and lungs to create body fluid while the 'dirty' part is passed down to the small intestine where it is again separated into pure and impure. On this occasion the pure portion goes to the bladder, the impure to the large intestine. The distribution of body fluid is mainly the task of the spleen through its function of 'transportation and transformation' and by the lung via its function of 'dispersing and descending'. Body fluid is part of blood, and so the liver and heart are both involved in the passage of body fluid, as is the kidney for excretion of urine.

Two types of pathology affects the body fluids, deficiency and accumulation (excess). Deficiency exists in such conditions as dry cough and dry mouth/tongue. Accumulation is seen in oedema and phlegm. Oedema is swelling as it is understood in western medicine, and phlegm is said to be fluid bubbles. Phlegm may exist in the lungs as in western medicine but also in other organs such as the heart where it gives rise to mental changes. The spleen, lungs and kidneys are involved with accumulation of body fluid. If these organs are deficient they cannot transform the body fluid. The fluid overflows from the channels and spills over into the space beneath the skin showing as oedema. The position of the oedema is important. That due to lung deficiency shows in the face and hands. Spleen deficiency oedema shows in the abdomen, and oedema due to kidney deficiency is seen in the legs and ankles (see page 17).

Clinical note

Clinically blood disorders are associated firstly with gynaecology and secondly skin disorders, reflecting either blood stasis or heat in the blood, respectively. The point SP-10 is called the 'sea of blood' and may be used in either of these cases, where it is said to 'cool the blood' and/or 'invigorate the blood'.

The eight principles

The eight principles are basic categories of syndromes which may be used to link a number of seemingly unconnected symptoms. The eight are yin/yang, exterior/interior, hot/cold, and deficiency/excess, and although described separately they are closely linked.

Yin and yang

The concept of yin and yang is central to all aspects of Chinese medicine. Yin indicates brightness while yang indicates darkness, the Chinese symbols for yin and yang literally meaning the 'sunny side of a hill' and a 'shady side of a hill'. Table 1.4 shows some of the correspondences to yin and yang. The basic concept of yin and yang is that everything in the universe follows an alternating cycle, e.g., day into night, growth into decay. Although each phenomenon is opposite, each also contains an aspect of the other. For example, day (yang) changes into night (yin); but as dawn breaks and the day proceeds, yang reaches a peak at mid-day and then starts to fade. At this point night (yin) begins to build up until by midnight day (yang) is at its minimum. As phenomena go through a continuous cycle, their form may also change cyclically. Thus the water in a lake evaporates into vapour only to come together as rain and drop back into the lake.

Table 1.4. Yin and yang correspondences.

Yang	Yin
Hot	Cold
Function	Substance
External	Internal
Light	Darkness
Sun	Moon
Activity	Rest
Heaven	Earth
Higher	Lower

Yin and yang are said to be in *mutual opposition*. In Table 1.4 we can see that hot is opposite to cold and light opposite to dark for example. At any time they each try to control one another, but by doing so they hold each other in check. Heat (yang) may dispel cold (yin) but equally cold may reduce heat. If both are equal, the temperature is normal. In the body there is a continual balance between yin and yang. If this balance is upset it will leave the other factor unrestrained. Yin is cool, and an excess of yin will make something colder. However a deficiency of yang (warm) will result in a proportional excess of yin and cold will still result.

Yin and yang depend on each other and are said to be *interdependent*. Yin represents the 'substance' and is said to be internal, while yang represents 'function' and is said to be external. To run (yang) one needs energy produced by digesting food (yin) but to digest food one needs digestive activity (yang). One cannot exist without the other and it is said that 'yang is the servant of yin and yin is the guard of yang' (Xinnong, 1999). The two aspects of yin and yang in any event are not fixed but are continually *consuming and producing* each other, a feature also known as 'waxing and waning'. As yin increases so yang reduces and vice versa. Under normal circumstances the two processes are in a state of balance, but if the balance is upset, too much of either yin or yang may be produced or consumed. Because yin and yang are intimately linked, there is an *inter-transforming* relationship between them. Extreme yin will change to yang and vice versa. In cases of high fever (yang) for example, the patient may begin to show signs of cold (yin) such as a drop in body temperature, pallor and a fading pulse. Yang has therefore transformed into yin. The clinical manifestations of yin and yang are shown in Table 1.5.

Table 1.5. Yin and yang clinical manifestations.

Yang	Yin
Acute disease	Chronic disease
Rapid onset	Gradual onset
Rapid pathological changes	Lingering
Heat	Cold
Restlessness and insomnia	Listlessness, sleeps well
Throws off bedclothes	Likes to be covered
Likes to stretch out	Likes to curl up
Hot body and limbs	Cold body and limbs
Red face	Pale face
Preference for cold drinks	Preference for hot drinks
Loud voice, talks a lot	Weak voice, dislikes talking
Coarse breathing	Shallow, weak breathing
Thirst	No thirst
Scanty, dark urine	Profuse, pale urine
Constipation	Loose stools
Red tongue with yellow coating	Pale tongue
Full pulse	Empty pulse

(From Maciocia, 1989)

Yin and yang are generally used to summarize the other six principles in clinical practice. Exterior, heat, and excess are yang in nature while interior, cold and deficiency are yin. In addition, yin and yang syndromes also exist as separate categories. A yin syndrome results from deficiency of yang qi and retention of pathogenic cold. Yang syndromes are caused by hyperactivity of yang qi and excess of pathogenic heat. Therefore deficiency/cold syndromes are yin and excess/heat syndromes are yang. Clinically, conditions characterized by fidgeting, hyperactivity and a bright (flushed) complexion are yang while those seen with inhibition, hypo-activity and a sallow complexion are yin (Xin and Jianping, 1994).

The position of a symptom is also associated with yin and yang. Body structures which are on the back or head, exterior or above the waist are yang while those which are on the front or body, interior or below the waist are yin (Table 1.6).

Table 1.6. Body structure position and yin–yang.

Yang	Yin
Back	Front
Head	Body
Exterior	Interior
Above the waist	Below the waist
Postero-lateral surface of limbs	Antero-medial surface of limbs
Fu organs	Zang organs
Organ function	Organ structure
Qi	Blood and body fluids
Defensive qi	Nutritive qi

(Maciocia, 1989)

The back and outside surfaces of the body are yang and have the function of protecting the body from pathogenic invasion. The front and inner surfaces are yin and have the function of nourishing the body. The yang channels all either start or finish on the head and so the head and body above the waist are said to be yang. In addition yang (heat) tends to rise upwards to the head. Equally, the head is easily affected by wind which is in itself yang. The body, especially below the waist is yin and is easily affected by the yin pathogenic factors cold and damp. The yang (fu) organs all transform, digest, or excrete 'impure' products while the yin (zang) organs store 'pure' essences. It is said that '*the 5 yin organs store but do not excrete, the 6 yang organs transform and digest but do not store*' (Simple questions, quoted in Maciocia, 1989).

Exterior and interior

The skin, hair, muscles and superficial portion of meridians and collaterals are described as external, while the Zang fu organs are internal. External conditions are said to be due to invasion of a superficial part of the body by a pathogen. These conditions have a sudden onset, with a short duration of symptoms. We can think here of the example of a 'cold' in the winter. The external conditions mainly show intolerance to cold and/or wind as their major feature. There is often a fever or 'temperature' and a thin tongue coating. The pulse feels superficial and faint, and is difficult to locate. The patient may complain of a headache and general aching with a blocked nose and a cough.

Invasion of external heat is distinguished from external cold by a number of features. With heat, the tongue coating is yellow while with cold the coating is white. In both cases the pulse is superficial, but with heat the heart rate is faster, described as a 'rapid pulse'. Invasion of external heat gives more severe fever and the patient becomes thirsty as the heat consumes fluid. Excess conditions do not give sweating while in deficiency conditions there is sweating as the skin pores are no longer controlled.

Interior syndromes occur through the transmission of a pathogen from the exterior to the interior to affect the Zang fu organs directly. There are three methods through which this may occur. Firstly an external pathogen may attack over a period of time, and the persistent nature of the pathogen overcomes the body's defenses to move internally. Secondly an external pathogen may also attack a Zang fu organ directly, and thirdly functional disturbances caused by emotional factors, improper diet, or physical/mental stress may weaken the body to such a degree that it is unable to repel the pathogen. In this case there is a deficiency (see below) of anti-pathogenic qi. In a similar way, a pathogenic factor may be transmitted from the interior to the exterior and expelled. This should occur with correct treatment as the anti-pathogenic qi is strengthened. It should also be pointed out that incorrect treatment may transmit an external pathogen to the interior! The outward transmission of pathogenic factors therefore indicates the remission of a disease; the inward transmission an exacerbation. For detail of transmission of an external pathogen in musculoskeletal conditions in particular see page 59.

Differentiating external from internal conditions is essentially a question of signs and symptoms and the stage of pathology. Fever (high temperature), accompanied by an aversion to cold suggests an external condition, while fever with no aversion to cold, or aversion to cold with no fever suggests an internal condition. The symptoms together therefore indicate an external condition, while the two occurring separately suggests an internal condition.

A thin white tongue coating possibly with red edges to the tongue suggests an external condition, while all other tongue changes indicate an internal (and more serious) pathology. A superficial pulse (easy to feel) is external, while a deep pulse (having to press hard to feel it) is internal.

Cold and hot

Cold and hot are manifestations of deficiency and excess of yin and yang. Cold is due to a predominance of yin, while hot is due to a predominance of yang. Cold syndromes are due to either an exposure to pathogenic cold or a deficiency of yang in the interior. The two conditions are opposite in nature. A patient exhibiting a cold syndrome will show a whitish complexion (pallor) and often demonstrate an aversion to cold. They will not drink great amounts of fluid but instead drink small amounts of hot drinks. There is generally an increased volume of fluid and the stools may be loose. The tongue coating is pale and moist and the pulse slow. In direct contrast the patient with heat will have a red complexion. They may have a fever and a thirst, with a preference for cold drinks. They show signs suggesting that body fluid is being consumed. The urine is scant and deep yellow in colour, and they may be constipated. The tongue is red often with a yellow dry coating and the pulse is rapid.

In cases of cold, moxibustion and warm needling are indicated together with retention of the needles for prolonged periods (reinforcing technique, see page 118) particularly of points such as ST-36 and CV-12. The stomach is said to dominate the Fu organs which are yang in nature. Using these points (CV-12 is the front Mu point of the stomach and the influential point of the Fu) will stimulate stomach function and create internal heat. In cases of heat these techniques would not be appropriate. Instead the excess heat is 'cleared' by swift needling (reduction method, see page 118) of points such as GV-14, LI-11 and LI-4. GV-14 is the 'sea of yang' and the meeting point of the yang channels with the governing vessel. It therefore has a marked effect on clearing pathogenic factors from the exterior. Both LI-4 and LI-11 are powerful at clearing heat. The lung channel (yin) is coupled to the large intestine (yang). As the lung controls the exterior (skin and hair), attack by an external pathogen may affect it first of all the organs. To use lung points would seem logical, but to do so poses the threat of allowing the pathogen to move to the interior if the wrong needling technique is used. Treating the large intestine as the coupled channel negates this threat.

Deficiency and excess

Deficiency and excess are terms used to describe the relationship between the strength of a pathogen and the proportional strength of anti-pathogenic qi. An *excess* condition exists when a pathogenic factor is hyperactive compared to normal anti-pathogenic qi. In contrast *deficiency* is present when anti-pathogenic qi is being consumed. Treatment will aim at either promoting anti-pathogenic qi in the case of deficiency, or eliminating the pathogenic factor in the case of excess.

Deficiency may be of either yin, yang, blood, or qi. Deficiency of yin gives heat symptoms while deficiency of yang gives cold symptoms. Deficiency of qi is seen after a long illness especially and shows as general lassitude. There may be spontaneous sweating due to the inability of qi to control the pores. Deficiency of blood is normally due to weakness in the spleen and stomach. Because blood is unable to reach the head the patient often experiences dizziness, and lack of blood to the heart may give palpitations.

General signs of deficiency include lassitude and weight loss, weak breathing, pallor, and night sweats. Where pain is present it is *alleviated by pressure* (see Chapter 4). The tongue is dry with little coating. Excess shows as agitation, rapid breathing, distension and fullness in the chest. Where pain is present it is *aggravated by pressure*. The tongue coating is thick and sticky.

The six pathogens

The six pathogens are wind, cold, summer heat, damp, dryness and fire (representing warmth and heat). Under normal circumstances these climatic changes do not pose a threat and are seen simply as six types of qi found in the natural environment (Xinnong, 1999). However, if the factors are particularly strong, or the change from one factor to another is sudden and unexpected, or if the body's ability to produce anti-pathogenic qi to combat the factors is weak, the pathogens can invade the body and cause harm. Each of the factors invades the exterior of the body (skin, mouth and nose) and may act in isolation or combination. In the case of musculoskeletal pain, the factors produce the bi syndromes (see page 54).

Wind is the main pathogen, as all the other pathogens depend on it for transport into the body. It is yang in nature and has two important characteristics in TCM. Firstly, wind is characterised by 'upward and outward dispersion' and is therefore likely to invade the upper part of the body and the external surface. Wind therefore attacks the head and face, and the lungs and skin. Secondly, wind by nature 'moves'. Conditions resulting from wind therefore show *movement* as part of their symptoms. Pains which change position, skin marking which appears and disappears, convulsions, spasms and tremors are all wind signs. Points such as GB-20 (wind pool), GV-16 (palace of wind), and BL-12 (wind gate) are used to treat wind-related conditions.

Cold is yin in nature, and is characterised by contraction and *stagnation*. Exposure to cold after sweating or when wearing thin clothing allows the cold to invade the body. Cold will consume the yang qi of the body and the warming function of the body is therefore impaired. Symptoms are cold limbs, stiffness, cold pain and contractions. There is a dislike of cold and lack of sweating. Treatment often involves moxibustion and warm needling, and reinforcing techniques.

Damp (a yin factor) occurs as a result of climate but also from damp rooms and exposure to wind in damp sweaty clothing. Damp is characterised by *heaviness*. Diseases caused by damp tend to be prolonged and show pain from obstruction of qi. There is poor body fluid dispersion resulting in oedema, and the tongue is swollen. Damp will affect the spleen and spleen points (especially SP-9 for oedema, and SP-6 for oedema of gynaecological origin) are often used to treat it.

Fire is a yang factor, with heat and then warmth milder forms of fire. Symptoms include *fever, thirst, headache, sweating* and *restlessness*. There is a rapid pulse and a red tongue. Yin fluid is consumed and dry lips, throat and mouth will result. Heat can in turn stir up wind which affects the liver. Reducing techniques are used when needling in the presence of fire.

Summer heat is not commonly seen in northern European countries. It occurs from over-exposure to the sun. Summer heat is yang in nature and the main symptoms are fever, *consumption of body fluids*, thirst, dizziness and lassitude.

Dryness affects the lung particularly. In invades through the mouth and nose and impairs the lung's function of 'moistening'. Signs include dry cough and sticky sputum.

The five elements

The five elements or 'five phases' is a method of linking and organising a variety of phenomena from nature and relating them clinically. The five elements are Fire, Earth, Metal, Water and Wood (Fig. 1.1). The five elements represent phases associated with movement or function. Wood is associated with the growing phase, fire with activity which has reached its peak and is about to decline. Metal represents function in decline while water represents function which has come to rest and is about to change directions. Earth represents neutrality or balance (Kaptchuk, 1983). The five elements can therefore be linked to the yin/yang system with wood and fire being the active (yang) phases, metal and water being the passive (yin) phases and water being the neutral phase which links yin to yang.

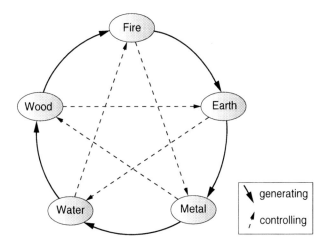

Figure 1.1. *Five element interrelationships*

The elements are arranged in a cycle with energy travelling around the cycle in a clockwise direction. This is known as the '*generating*' or interpromoting aspect of the cycle. If we take the element fire as an example it promotes earth (the next element in the cycle) and earth promotes metal. We have simply followed the direction of the curved arrows. This interpromoting characteristic is known as the 'mother–son' relationship. Fire is the mother (the producer) of earth while metal is the son (the produced) of earth. This has a direct relationship to acupuncture point selection where mother and son points are used to tonify and sedate the energy within a meridian (see page 69).

In addition to the arrows passing around the circumference of the cycle, there are arrows passing across the cycle. This portion of the cycle is known as '*controlling*' or interacting. Following the direction of the straight arrows it can be seen that Fire controls metal and is controlled by water. Any change in one element therefore affects the others.

The zang fu organs are attributed to each element (Fig. 1.2 and Table 1.7) and in addition each element has a taste, colour, emotion, and tissue associated with it. Clinically the five element theory may be used to link seemingly disparate symptoms. For example, a patient with eye problems and muscle tremors which increase at times of anger may be seen to be linked by the element wood. This element relates to liver and over-activity of the liver may be calmed both by using the sedation point (son point, LR-2) and also by tonifying the lung or large intestine meridians.

Table 1.7. Five element correspondences.

Element	Zang	Fu	Sense organ	Tissue	Emotion	Taste	Colour
Wood	Liver	Gallbladder	Eye	Tendon	Anger	Sour	Green
Fire	Heart	Small intestine	Tongue	Vessel	Joy	Bitter	Red
Earth	Spleen	Stomach	Mouth	Muscle	Worry	Sweet	Yellow
Metal	Lung	Large intestine	Nose	Skin and hair	Grief and melancholy	Pungent	White
Water	Kidney	Bladder	Ear	Bone	Fear	Salty	Black

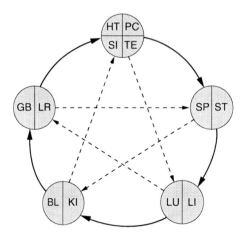

Figure 1.2. *Five element Zang Fu*

The Zang Fu organs

The Zang Fu organs are central to the whole concept of traditional Chinese medicine (TCM) and as such are vital to the workings of traditional Chinese acupuncture. In western acupuncture the Zang Fu organs are of less importance, but an understanding of the basic functions of the Zang Fu organs helps the practitioner to decide on appropriate acupuncture points to needle.

The names given to the Zang Fu organs refer to functions attributed to the organs by the ancient Chinese. The ancient Chinese did not place great emphasis on structure and never used dissection. Through observation they discovered the basic physiological functions of the heart and digestive tract for example, but attributed many other functions to the Zang Fu which are unfamiliar to the western medical practitioner. Unfortunately the names given in the west to the Zang Fu organs are those also used for the organs themselves. This leads to confusion as the names used by the ancient Chinese normally only refer to an observed body function rather than to an organ structure. The Zang Fu are often referred to as 'functional systems' rather than organs, to differentiate them from the traditional use of the word 'organ' in western medicine.

Table 2.1. The Zang Fu organs.

Zang	Fu
Yin	Yang
Solid	Hollow
Processing products	Storage
Heart	Small intestine
Lungs	Large intestine
Liver	Gallbladder
Spleen	Stomach
Kidney	Bladder
(Pericardium)	Triple energiser

There are six Fu organs which are yang in nature and five Zang organs which are yin in nature (Table 2.1). The Fu organs are hollow and principally used for storage whereas the Zang organs are solid and used mainly for processing products. The functions of the Fu organs are similar to those given to these organs in the west, but the functions of the Zang are somewhat more complex.

The Zang organs

Heart *Xin*

The heart (Table 2.2) is considered in TCM the most important of all the organs and is sometimes referred to as 'the monarch of all organs'. As with all organs the structure (of the heart, blood vessels and blood) consisting of matter is considered yin. The function, consisting of energy is considered yang. The heart controls the blood circulation and is said to 'dominate the blood vessels'. Heart qi is the driving force behind the heartbeat itself and the strength, rate and rhythm of the heartbeat will all be affected if the heart qi is weak. Changes in both the heart qi and the heart blood will show in the pulse. Deficiency will show as a weak pulse in general, and deficiency of heart qi/blood will show as weakness in the distal pulse position of the left hand (see page 104). Transformation of food qi into blood is said to take place in the heart and so the heart has the function not just of propelling the blood but actually creating it in TCM.

Table 2.2. Heart *Xin* (the monarch of all organs).

Dominates the blood vessels.
Manifests in the face.
Houses the mind.
Opens to the tongue.

In TCM the heart also has a primary function in mental activities. This function is not seen in western medicine but is obvious in poetry for example. It is interesting to note that mental problems such as stress and anxiety are seen as a prime cause of heart disease in the west and some complementary practitioners are calling for a new approach to 'healing the heart' using meditation, for example, to take a spiritual approach to reversing coronary artery disease (Chopra, 1998). This approach is very much in line with the traditional Chinese view of the heart system. If the heart is functioning correctly the patient will have sound mental activity and healthy vigour. If the heart is functioning poorly the patient may show mental disturbance and eventually even insanity. The heart organ is related to sleep, and heart points such as HT-7 are frequently used in the treatment of insomnia. It is said that if the heart is weak, 'the mind will have no residence' and will float at night causing excessive dreaming or disturbed sleep.

Sweat is said to be a heart fluid. The logic behind this is that sweat comes from body fluid, and the main constituent of body fluid in TCM is said to be blood. It is said that 'blood and sweat have the same source' and that sweat comes from the 'space between the skin and muscles'. Deficiency of heart qi causes the patient to lose control of the sweating process and spontaneous sweating occurs. Similarly sweating is a sign of excess yang in the heart while deficiency of yin, which will give a proportional excess of yang, can cause night sweating.

Finally, the heart has a strong connection with the ability to speak, and changes in the way a patient speaks may be diagnostic of heart system disorders. The tongue is said to be 'the sprout of the heart' and the tongue body comes from a branch of the heart meridian. The tongue itself may be pale if the heart is insufficient or blue in cases of blood stagnation. A central crack in the tongue shows weakness in the heart and a red tip shows heat. The face also has a relation to the heart. The face has a rich supply of blood vessels and so if the heart is healthy the patient will have a rosy complexion. Paleness in the face is said to show deficiency while a blue tinge shows stagnation.

Case history

A busy career woman with a hectic lifestyle was suffering from recurrent nightmares which were gradually increasing over the last five years. On average they occurred three times per week. Each time she had a nightmare she woke sweating profusely, feeling hot, with a desire to throw the bedclothes off. She had a history of constipation and dizziness. The pulse was forceful and superficial, with the heart and lung levels fainter. The tongue was slightly swollen with noticeable tooth marks, and the tip of the tongue was red. The clinical picture suggests an excess pattern of heat, most likely heart phlegm.

Point selection

ST-40 to clear phlegm from the heart and calm the spirit.
SP-6 to resolve phlegm.
HT-5 luo connecting point of the heart, to calm the spirit.
HT-7 yuan source point to calm the spirit and regulate the heart.
GV-20 to subdue yang and benefit the head.

Lung *Fei*

The lung (Table 2.3) is said in TCM to be the most external organ, sometimes called the 'canopy of the body'. Being the most external it is the organ most susceptible to invasion by external pathogens such as cold and wind. The nose is known as the 'gateway to the lungs' and as it leads to the larynx the voice is often affected in lung conditions. The lung is said to house the corporeal soul (see page 16) and so it is easily affected by grief and sadness, especially when this has been caused by bereavement.

Clinical note

The soul or spirit in TCM is divided into the 'corporeal soul' housed in the lung and the ethereal soul housed in the liver. The corporeal soul is the physical manifestation of the spirit, inseparably linked to the body, which returns to the earth upon death. The ethereal soul is that part of the spirit which survives after death to enter a world of subtle non-material energies (Maciocia, 1989) and is the more literal translation of the western term 'soul'. The corporeal soul is closely related to breathing and it can be said to be the 'breath of life' housed in the lungs. It is affected by the emotions of sadness and grief especially, particularly when brought on by bereavement. These emotions are said to restrict the corporeal soul and reduce lung qi giving shallow apical type breathing. Treatment is to needle LU-7 to release the emotions and BL-42 the 'door of the corporeal soul'. Needling LU-7 can cause the patient with repressed emotions to cry, weeping being the sound made by the lung according to 5 element thinking. BL-42 is level with BL-13 (back shu point of the lung) but on the outer bladder line. Needling BL-42 aims to cause the lung qi to descend and to soothe the spirit.

Table 2.3. Lung *Fei* (the most external organ of the body).

Dominates qi.
Controls respiration.
Dominates dispersing and descending.
Dominates skin and hair.
Regulates the water passages.
Opens to the nose.

The lung both dominates qi and controls respiration. The lung is the organ through which qi of the exterior and interior mingle. Clear qi is inhaled and waste qi is exhaled. Pectoral qi (Zong qi) is formed by combining the essential parts of water and food with the clear qi inhaled by the lung. The pectoral qi accumulates in the chest and then ascends to the larynx and is distributed throughout the body via the heart meridian. Any deficiency in the lung qi will therefore obstruct this passage and lead to lassitude, weak speech, weak respiration and shortness of breath.

Case history

This patient had a history of annual hay fever. His eyes were red and his nose running. The tongue was of normal size with a sticky white coating. The tongue tip was redder than normal. The patient had no audible wheeze and showed no difficulty in breathing. The patient was a student who regularly suffered from hay fever each year from June/July to September/October. His symptoms were made worse when the pollen count was high and especially when he was near cut grass. There was slight blockage to the frontal and maxillary sinuses which was exacerbated to pressure. Pulse examination showed a superficial, rapid, bounding pulse.
The clinical picture suggested invasion of wind heat with deficiency of the lung and failure to disperse/descend.

Point selection

GB-21 to disperse wind.
LU-7 to strengthen the lung.
LI-4 general point for all head conditions.
LI-11 to expel wind.
Yintang (extra) to disperse phlegm in the nose.
LI-20 to disperse phlegm in the nose.

The lung dominates dispersing and also dominates the skin and hair. The lung is said to distribute defensive qi and body fluids to the whole body and to warm and moisten the tissues. Body fluids are distributed in the form of a fine mist and the skin, hair and sweat glands on the body surface act as a protective screen against external pathogens. In TCM it is said that 'the pores are the gate of qi' meaning both that the defensive qi passes through the pores onto the skin surface, but also that external pathogens may enter the body through the pores if the defensive qi is deficient. These pathogens then enter the lung (hence the lung is referred to as the most external organ) giving rise to aversion to cold, fever, obstruction and cough.

The lung is also said to dominate descending and to regulate the water passages. The qi of the upper Zang Fu organs descends while that of the lower organs ascends. Lung qi is therefore meant to descend but if it does not, upward perversion of lung qi can cause stuffiness in the chest accompanied by shortness of breath and cough. Again, regulation of the water passages depends on the lung's descending function. Pure water from food is passed from the spleen and stomach to the lungs. Some is dispersed to the skin and muscles and some (the impure portion) sent to the kidney and bladder. If the descending function of the lung is impaired, fluid will be retained as phlegm or oedema.

The lung is said to 'open to the nose', with both respiration and olfaction depending on lung qi. If the lung is functioning correctly respiration is free and the sense of smell acute. Poor function with deficiency of lung qi leads to nasal obstruction and a runny nose. The throat is said to be the gateway of respiration and as it also houses the organs of speech, disorders of speech are often treated using lung points. Changes in lung qi can lead to a hoarse voice or loss of the voice in some cases, and points such as LU-7 and LI-4 may be used (both command points and heavenly star points) as the lung channel is internally–externally linked to the large intestine channel.

Spleen *Pi*

The spleen (Table 2.4) is the central organ of the digestive system and is linked to the stomach. It is concerned with fluid balance, and the ability of spleen points to treat oedema is particularly important in musculoskeletal therapy.

> **Clinical note**
>
> Swelling may be treated by using either lung, spleen (supported by the stomach), or kidney points. Dysfunction in any or these organs will impair fluid transformation. This may lead to an overflow of fluid from the meridian channels into the space between the skin and muscles to form oedema. Fluid may also overflow to form phlegm, either settling in the lungs or in the meridian channels where it can cause obstruction. Where oedema is in the upper part of the body, especially in the face and hands, lung points are used. When the oedema is spread across the middle portion of the body, spleen points are more effective. Oedema of the lower limbs, especially swollen feet and ankles responds better to needling bladder points.
>
> Spleen points may be used to transform any type of phlegm, with lung points supplementing them for phlegm associated with cough and sputum production. ST-40 is possibly the most important point to use in the treatment of phlegm. It is the luo connecting point with the spleen.

Table 2.4. Spleen *Pi* (the central organ of the digestive system).

Governs transportation and transformation.
Controls the blood.
Dominates the muscles and the four limbs.
Opens to the mouth.
Manifests in the lips.

The spleen is said to 'govern transportation and transformation' and is responsible for digestion and the transmission and absorption of nutrient substances in TCM. Food is taken into the stomach and digested by both the stomach and the spleen. As food is the basis of qi formation after birth, the spleen is considered the main organ for manufacturing both blood and qi. Deficiency of the spleen may lead to poor appetite, abdominal distension and malnutrition in extreme cases.

Case history

A young female patient showed regular tiredness and lack of energy with poor concentration. She had no appetite and suffered from occasional diarrhoea. Her eating habits were erratic and her diet generally poor. Her tongue was pale and slightly swollen. Her pulse was faint. The patient's complexion was pale and her lips were dry and cracked. The picture suggests deficiency of the spleen.

Point selection

ST-36 to tonify qi and harmonise the stomach.
SP-3 source point.
SP-6 tonify the spleen and stomach.
BL-20 back shu point of the spleen.
BL-21 back shu point of the stomach.

The spleen has an important role in water metabolism and is said to transport and transform dampness. It ensures that the tissues are adequately moistened but at the same time free from retention of dampness in the form of either phlegm or oedema. As a lower Zang Fu organ, the spleen qi should ascend, if it descends the clinical manifestation can be vertigo, blurred vision or prolapse.

The spleen has the function of controlling the blood. By this it is meant that the spleen acts to keep the blood within the blood vessels. If spleen qi is deficient blood can escape (extravasation) and may appear as bruising, blood in the stools or urine, or uterine bleeding. The spleen is therefore an organ particularly involved with gynaecological disorders. The spleen is said to dominate the muscles and the four limbs, in that it nourishes the muscles and enhances their bulk. Food qi is extracted by the stomach and sent to the muscles by the spleen. If the spleen qi is deficient the patient is likely to feel weak and muscle wasting may occur in extreme cases.

The spleen is said to open to the mouth and manifest in the lips. The spleen function is closely related to food intake and the sense of taste. If the patient suffers from spleen dysfunction, the appetite may be poor and the sense of taste impaired. There may also be a sticky sweet taste in the mouth. Because the mouth is said to be the aperture of the spleen the lips will reflect the spleen condition. Normally the lips should be red and lustrous but in cases of spleen deficiency the lips may be pale and sallow.

The spleen together with the heart and kidney has a direct effect on our mental processes. The spleen is said to be the residence of thought and is important for activities, such as studying, which require concentration. The heart is said to house the mind and is important for long-term memory and thought processes which effect life events. The kidney is said to nourish the brain and is responsible for short-term memory and day to day basic activities.

Liver *Gan*

The main function of the liver (Table 2.5) is storing blood and it is an important organ (together with the spleen) in the treatment of menstrual problems. In storing blood, the liver alters blood volume between exercise and rest, for example. Any disease of the liver may lead to blood disease itself, a factor in many skin conditions. The liver is said to maintain the free flow of qi. It is an organ which dislikes depression and is readily affected by emotional changes in general. These may cause liver qi stagnation (often seen in headaches). The liver is said to open to the eye. It is said that 'tears are the fluid of the liver', and it is interesting to note that many headaches, (migraine especially), are accompanied by eye pain, watering of the eye or partial closure of the eyelid. These conditions are often effectively treated by needling LR-3. The liver function of maintaining the free flow of qi is related to the digestive processes of the stomach and spleen. Because of this liver qi stagnation may cause a reciprocal effect on the stomach giving nausea and vomiting.

Table 2.5. Liver *Gan* (governs the body like a general controlling an army).

Stores blood.
Maintains the free flow of qi.
Controls the tendons.
Manifest in the nails.
Opens to the eye.

Case history

A young female patient had experienced headaches each week for the last one year, focussed over the right eye. When the headache was present the right eye was red and partially closed and the patient experienced mild photophobia. During this time, the patient wanted to place her head on a cool pillow. Anxiety made the headaches worse. The patient's pulse was normal and the tongue showed a slightly purplish discoloration. The clinical picture suggested an excess of yang, especially in the liver.

Point selection

LR-3 (source point) to subdue liver yang.
ST-36 general point to calm the spirit.
LL-4 general point for head symptoms.
SP-6 to harmonise the liver.
Taiyang (extra) right side only (tender to palpation).

The liver controls the tendons (sinews) and manifests in the nails. If liver blood is consumed it may deprive the tendons of nourishment, giving rise to weakness. If the tendons are invaded by pathogenic heat, this may result in convulsions. The liver therefore controls muscle action and muscle tone (function) whereas the spleen controls muscle bulk (structure). The nails are said to be the 'surplus of tendons' and so the liver manifests in the nails and changes in the nail bed or nail itself may be seen in cases of severe liver dysfunction. Typical changes include darkening, dryness and cracking.

The liver meridian connects to the eye and the liver organ is said to open to the eye. Liver deficiency may therefore lead to dryness of the eyes, blurred vision or even night blindness. Excess heat (yang) in the liver may give redness, swelling and pain in the eyes, again often seen with certain types of headaches which may be helped by using LR-3 or BL-18 (back shu point of the liver) as two of the points.

Kidney *Shen*

The kidney (Table 2.6) is said to be the root of life and it is responsible for storing the essence. Kidney yin is said to be the fundamental substance (structure) of birth and growth, while kidney yang is the motive force (function). The kidney therefore dominates both reproduction and development. Kidney essence may be either congenital (from parents) or acquired (from essential substances transformed by the spleen and stomach). Essence is said to follow a seven year cycle for women, and an eight year cycle for men. Essence flourishes at age 14 in females and declines at age 49. In males it flourishes at 16 and declines at age 56 and is finally gone at age 64. Kidney yin is the foundation of all yin fluids in the body which moisten the Zang Fu organs. If kidney yin is deficient it will fail to control kidney yang and symptoms are heat in the chest, palms and soles, night sweats and seminal emission. If kidney yang is deficient, leading to a failure of warming and promoting, there will be coldness and pain in the lumbar region, and possibly impotence.

Table 2.6. Kidney *Shen* (the root of life).

Stores essence.
Dominates reproduction and development.
Dominates water metabolism.
Receives the qi.
Dominates bone.
Manufactures marrow to fill the brain.
Manifests in the hair.
Opens to the ear.
Dominates anterior and posterior orifices.

The kidney is said to dominate water metabolism. Water is received by the stomach and then transmitted by the spleen to the lung, which disperses and descends it. Part of the fluid reaches the kidney where it is divided into clear and turbid (unclean) portions. The clear portion goes to the lung to be circulated to the organs and tissues. The turbid portion goes to the bladder to form urine. If the kidney fails to open and close one of the results will be oedema and/or abnormal micturition.

The kidney is said to receive the qi, and works with the lung in this function. It is said that 'the lung is the governor of qi and the kidney is the root of qi'. The lung receives the clear qi from the air and passes it down to the kidney which holds it. Kidney qi must be strong for the passage of qi to be free and for respiration to be smooth. If kidney qi is weak (deficient), the root of qi is not firm and the kidney will fail to hold the qi, giving shortness of breath especially on exertion. This is often seen in chronic asthma (also called deficiency-type asthma in TCM), for example, where lung points (LU-9 or BL-13, back shu point of the lung) and kidney points (KI-3) may be combined.

Case history

An elderly, frail patient presented with long-standing asthma. She had a slightly stooped appearance with a flattened anterior chest suggesting a history of breathing difficulties. Her tongue examination revealed a normal tongue body with a thin white coating. The tongue was larger than normal giving the appearance of filling the mouth, and there were a number of lateral cracks on either side of the tongue. The patient described dryness of her throat with a desire to drink, especially during the evening and at night. The patient woke two or three times at night to go to the toilet. The urine was clear with no recent change in volume. The patient's sleep was disturbed by palpitations, and she was breathless on exertion.

To palpation, the chest was quite rigid with poor expansion. Breathing was isolated to the upper regions. Pulse examination showed a deep slippery pulse with the lung level weak and the kidney level moderately weak.

This clinical picture shows deficiency. The history and pulse suggest deficiency in the lung and kidney. The aim of treatment is to tonify the lung and kidney, and release the tightness in the chest.

Point selection

CV-17 major point for asthma/wheezing and local point to chest symptoms.
Dingchuan, extra point (0.5 cun lateral to GV-14) major point for asthma and wheezing.
HT-7 (source point) to reduce palpitations.
PC-6 (luo connecting point) to unbind the chest and reduce palpitations.
KI-3 (source point) to nourish the kidney and benefit the lung.
BL-23 shu point of kidney.
BL-13 shu point of the lung.
SP-6 swelling in the ankle.

An important feature of the kidney with respect to musculoskeletal treatment is that of dominating bone. The kidney is said to manufacture marrow to fill the brain. Marrow in this context consists of two parts, bone marrow and spinal marrow. Spinal marrow ascends to the brain and it is said that 'the brain is the sea of marrow'. Bone marrow develops in the bone cavities and nourishes the bones. If the kidney essence is deficient bones will not be nourished and the patient may get soreness in the lumbar region, knees, and feet and possibly maldevelopment. Teeth are the 'surplus of bone' and kidney deficiency may ultimately lead to loss of teeth.

The kidney manifests in the hair. Hair is said to be the 'surplus of blood'. Hair nourishment depends on the blood, but its vitality depends on the kidney. Hair loss and lustre both depend on the health of the kidney. In the prime of life hair is lustrous, as kidney qi declines however the hair turns white and eventually falls out.

The kidney opens to the ears and hearing relies on nourishment of the kidney by essential qi. If essential qi is deficient, it will not ascend to the ear and tinnitus and deafness may result. This is why kidney points such as KI-3 and BL-23 (back shu point of the kidney) are often used in the treatment of tinnitus. The kidney also dominates the anterior and posterior orifices. The anterior orifice (urethra and genitalia) and posterior orifice (anus) rely on kidney qi activity for function. Deficiency may give impotence, disorders of micturition and prolapse.

The Fu organs

The Fu organs themselves (Table 2.7) are generally less important clinically than the Zang, but their meridian pathways are often used in the treatment of musculoskeletal conditions. Gallbladder (Dan) function is closely related to the liver. The gallbladder stores bile and continuously excretes it to the intestines. In normal function gallbladder qi descends. Upward perversion of gallbladder qi gives rise to a bitter taste in the mouth and failure to aid the stomach and spleen resulting in abdominal distension and loose stools. The gallbladder is closely related to the liver's function in maintaining the free flow of qi. In addition it shares the liver's relation to emotional changes and can be associated with fear and dreaming. The gallbladder is sometimes called an extra Fu organ. This is because it manufactures a substance rather than receiving water and food like the other Fu organs.

Table 2.7. The Fu organs.

Organ	Basic function
Gallbladder	Stores bile
Stomach	Receives and decomposes food
Small intestine	Separates the clear from the turbid
Large intestine	Receives waste from the small intestine, absorbs fluid and forms the remainder into faeces
Bladder	Temporary storage of urine
Triple energiser	Passage for Yuan qi

The stomach (Wei) is related to the spleen, and together these two are the most important of the Fu organs as they are said to be the 'root of post heaven qi', that is they produce blood and qi from food. The stomach receives and decomposes food and then transmits it to the small intestine. Essential substances are transported and transformed by the spleen. The stomach and spleen are therefore the main organs carrying out digestion and absorption and together they are known as the 'acquired foundation'. If the descending function of the stomach is disturbed, there is a lack of appetite and distending pain in the epigastrium with possible nausea and vomiting.

The small intestine (Xiaochang) is related to the heart. Its main function is to receive food from the stomach and further digest it. The stomach is said to 'separate the clear from the turbid', absorbing the essential substances and some water, and transmitting the food residue to the large intestine and the water residue to the bladder. Dysfunction of the small intestine affects digestion, but can also affect bowel movement and urination. The large intestine (Dachang) communicates with the lung. It receives waste material from the small intestine, absorbs the fluid content and forms the rest into faeces for excretion. Dysfunction may result in constipation or loose stools. In terms of musculoskeletal treatment, the pathway of the large intestine meridian and that of the triple energiser over the shoulder is especially important to shoulder conditions.

Case history

A patient presented with shoulder pain to abduction with a positive Hawkins sign confirming gleno-humeral impingement. Pain was produced with resisted lateral rotation and abduction of the humerus suggesting the supraspinatus muscle as the impinged structure. Shoulder extension was slightly painful and pain was experienced across the front and side of the shoulder and down the arm as far as the elbow. Tongue examination showed a normal red tongue body with a thin white coating and slight red edges suggesting an external syndrome. The pulse was superficial and forceful. The pain was generally eased by heat and in hot weather and was worse in cold weather. Bladder and bowel habits were normal. Movement eased stiffness and pain providing it was below the horizontal position of the shoulder.
The clinical picture suggests a deficiency syndrome with obstruction in the large intestine and triple energiser meridians giving shoulder symptoms.

Point selection

ST-38 distal point, needled while the patient attempted to move the shoulder. Pain was eased and range of motion gradually increased.
LI-15 local point for shoulder pain.
TE-14 local point for shoulder pain.
Jianqian (extra point) for anterior shoulder pain.
LI-11 as the mother point of the large intestine meridian.
LI-4 (source point) for pain relief.

The bladder (Pang Guang) is connected to the kidney. It temporarily stores urine which is discharged from the body through qi activity. This process is assisted by (and dependent upon) kidney qi. Dysfunction may lead to incontinence, frequency or dysuria. In the treatment of musculoskeletal conditions the path of the bladder channel, and its relation to low back pain, is more important than the bladder organ itself. The relationship between the bladder channel position and the kidney organ function of dominating the bones is especially important in cases of chronic low back pain.

Case history

A patient presented with a history of right-sided sciatica for seven months. The pain was referred to the posterior thigh, posterior calf and into the ankle. The patient felt better when warm, and his symptoms were increased in cold damp weather and eased by heat. Urine and stools had not changed noticeably in consistency but the patient woke twice at night needing to pass water. Tongue examination revealed a red tongue body with a sticky peeling coating. The coating was slightly white. Pulse diagnosis revealed a deep pulse with the kidney region very faint.

This picture shows invasion of cold and damp into the bladder and kidney meridians. The aim of treatment is to warm the qi and to resolve pain.

Point selection

KI-3 right side only. To strengthen the kidney.

BL-60 (heavenly star point). To activate entire channel. May be joined by through needling to KI-3.

BL-40 right side only. To activate the channel and benefit the lumbar region.

BL-23 bilateral. Back shu of the kidney.

GB-30 right side only. Local point for sciatic pain referred into the outer buttock.

The Triple Energiser (Sanjiao) is related to the pericardium. It governs various forms of qi and acts as a passage for the flow of yuan qi (original qi) from the kidney. The Triple Energiser is divided into upper (above diaphragm), middle (between diaphragm and umbilicus) and lower (below umbilicus) regions or 'jiao' each related to Zang Fu organs in these regions. It is said that the 'upper jiao is like a fog', and assists the heart and lung. 'The middle jiao looks like a froth of bubbles' and assists the spleen and stomach in decomposing food. 'The lower jiao looks like a drainage ditch', and helps the kidney, bladder and large intestine.

Meridians

General outline

The meridians and their collaterals are said to be the pathways through which qi (and blood) circulate. Traditionally, the meridians have been likened to the main trunk of a tree while the collaterals are compared to the branches. The roots are said to be represented by the Zang Fu organs while the flowers are the sense organs. Damage to the roots will therefore affect the trunk and branches and show in the flowers (sense organs, especially the tongue).

The meridians travelling on the inner aspects of the limb are known as yin meridians, those on the outer aspects of the limb as yang meridians. The yin meridians connect with Zang organs, while the yang meridians connect with the Fu organs (see Chapter 2). The three yin meridians of the arm (lung, heart and pericardium) all begin on the chest and travel to the hand. The three yang meridians of the arm (large intestine, small intestine and Triple Energiser) begin on the hand and travel to the head. The three yin meridians of the leg (spleen, liver and kidney) begin on the foot and travel along the inner aspect of the leg to the torso. The three yang meridians of the leg (bladder, gallbladder and stomach) begin on the face, near the eye, and travel down to the foot. All the yang meridians therefore start and finish in the head (Fig. 3.1).

The meridians form a continuous network of external and internal pathways. The external pathways or 'primary channels' are those represented on standard acupuncture charts, and it is the external pathway which contains the acupuncture points. The internal pathway is also important although it cannot be seen. The internal pathways consist of a number of branches which connect the meridians to the Zang Fu organs and also form connections between the various meridians themselves. An appreciation of the internal pathways is useful to explain the sometimes puzzling relationship between acupuncture points and symptoms. Needling a point on a channel will target local symptoms such as pain, but can also treat the organs to which a meridian is directly or indirectly connected.

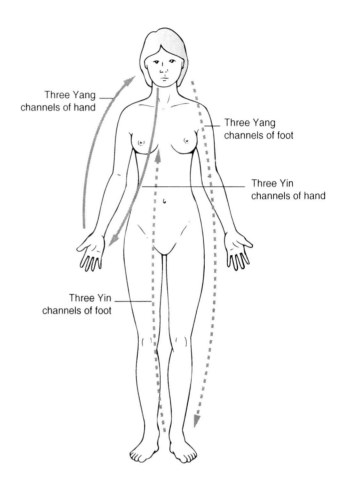

Three Yang channels of hand

Three Yang channels of foot

Three Yin channels of hand

Three Yin channels of foot

Figure 3.1. *General position of the 12 regular meridians. (Reproduced with permission from Hopwood et al., 1997)*

The external meridians form three interconnected circuits (Table 3.1a). The yin meridians flow to the yang meridians. This relationship is called *internal-external pairing*, the yin channels of the arm being paired with a yang arm channel and each yin channel of the leg being paired with a yang leg channel. This pairing represents not just the channel pairing, but the pairing of each of the Zang organs with a Fu organ. Similarly, each of the yin channels of the arm is paired to a yin channel of the leg, and the same is true of the yang channels. It is as though the two channels were really one, and as a consequence this is called the *six channel pairing*, there being six pairs of meridians in the 12 regular series. Rather than the Zang Fu relationship, the six channel pairing relies on anatomical position. For example, in normal standing with the arms by the sides, the large intestine meridian (yang) is anterior in the arm. In the same standing position, the meridian linked to it in the six channel pairing, the stomach (yang), lies in an anterior position in the leg.

The six channel pairing also represents levels of energy within the meridian system. With the small intestine and bladder meridians (Tai Yang or Major Yang) being the most exterior of the yang meridians. The sequence is shown in Table 3.1b.

The circulation of qi begins in the yin channel in the chest (on the first circuit this is the lung) and travels to the interiorly–exteriorly related yang channel on the hand (large intestine). The flow is then to the face to the six channel paired yang meridian on the leg (stomach) where the qi descends to the foot to pass to the interiorly–exteriorly paired yin channel (spleen) to return to the chest and begin its circulation in the second circuit yin channel (heart).

Table 3.1a. Meridian circuits.

	Yin	*Yang*	*Yang*	*Yin*
1st circuit	Lung	Large intestine	Stomach	Spleen
2nd circuit	Heart	Small intestine	Bladder	Kidney
3rd circuit	Pericardium	Triple Energiser	Gallbladder	Liver

Table 3.1b. Depth of meridian pairs.

	Pinyin Name	*English Name*	*Meridians*
Exterior	Tai yang	Major yang	SI & BL
	Shao yang	Minor yang	TE & GB
	Yang ming	Brilliant yang	LI & ST
	Tai yin	Major yin	SP & LU
	Jue yin	Absolute yin	LR & PC
	Shao yin	Minor yin	KI & HT

The internal channels consist of the 12 divergent channels, the 15 luo-connecting vessels, and the internal portions of the eight extraordinary meridians. The divergent channels branch from the main channels and have no separate points themselves. The divergent channels form a further connection between the main meridian channels and their related Zang Fu organs, and connect areas of the body not supplied by the external channels themselves. In particular they increase the distribution of qi and blood to the head. Not all of the meridian external channels travel to the head but the divergent channels provide a connection between the external channels of the yin meridians in particular and the head. The luo-connecting vessels lie superficially on the body (see Fig. 3.2). There is one luo-connecting vessel for each of the 12 regular meridians as well as one each for the CV and GV meridians. In addition the spleen has a second luo channel, 'the great luo-connecting channel of the spleen'. The luo-connecting channels leave the primary channel at the luo points (see Table 5.5, page 67) to connect their internally–externally related meridian pair. After joining their paired channel, many luo channels follow their own individual path as detailed below.

The meridians are said to lie at specific depths (Pirog, 1996). The cutaneous regions and meridian sinews lie directly beneath the skin (Fig. 3.2). Immediately beneath these lie the luo-connecting vessels and then the main meridian itself. The extraordinary vessel lies deep to the main meridian, nearest to the bone.

Although attempts have been made to find a specific anatomical structure which forms the meridian, the idea that meridians have a single material form is generally not accepted (James, 1993). The more

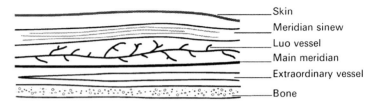

Figure 3.2. *The depths of the meridians. (Reproduced with permission from Pirog, 1996)*

likely case is that the meridians represent a functional link between the acupuncture points and exist as areas of influence over certain sections of the body (Maciocia, 1989). It is thought that a number of anatomical structures contribute to give meridians their characteristics. Physical transmission may occur along meridians through a combination of ionic movement inside the interstitial spaces and neurotransmission within neurovascular bundles (Wei et al., 1999).

Meridian function

The meridians have several functions. Firstly they are said to transport qi and blood. Nutrient qi is said to flow inside the meridians to be transported to the body tissues and organs while defensive qi is said to run outside the main meridian channel. The meridians form an interweaving network transporting qi and blood throughout the body, nourishing, warming and energising all the tissues. Secondly, the meridians resist pathogenic attack upon the body, but in so doing will show signs and symptoms of illness and disease themselves. In traditional Chinese medicine inspection of the skin and inspection of the tongue in particular is an important method of assessing the patient. For example the liver is said to be 'open to the eye' and 'manifest in the nails' while the kidney 'opens to the ear' and 'manifests in the hair'. Changes in these sites can therefore be diagnostic in themselves, with the channels reflecting disease within the Zang Fu organs. Because the meridians connect the Zang Fu organs, disease may also be transmitted between the organs via the meridian channels. When the body is under attack by a pathogen, it is the function of the meridians to contain the pathogen and prevent penetration into the body. Because the meridians lie at different levels the outer levels (sinew channels) will be attacked first by an external pathogen followed by the collaterals and primary channels. When the pathogen gets past the deepest levels it will enter the Zang Fu organs and cause severe harm.

The third property of meridians is the transmission of sensation along the channel. Stimulation of an acupuncture point is said to affect its relevant organ with the aim of restoring the free flow of blood and qi. Needling methods are used to reinforce (increase) or reduce (decrease) the flow of energy through a meridian. The outward manifestation of this being achieved is the sensation of Deqi (arrival of qi) which is often described as a deep ache which begins local to the needled point and travels away from it both proximally and distally. Some patients describe tingling, or a sensation of water flowing or warmth. Methods of obtaining the Deqi sensation are described on page 113.

The main outpatient symptoms associated with the 12 regular meridians are shown in Table 3.2.

Table 3.2. Main outpatient symptoms associated with the 12 primary meridians.

Meridian	Main symptoms
Lung	Nasal congestion, cough, wheezing and dyspnoea. Fullness in the chest, expectoration. Pain in the supraclavicular fossa, chest, shoulders and back. Cold pain along the anterior aspect of the arm. Headache.
Large intestine	Shoulder and upper arm pain. Toothache. Pain and redness of the eyes. Sore throat. Lower abdominal pain.
Stomach	Pain in the anterior leg. Pain in the eyes. Nosebleed. Lesions of the lips and mouth. Abdominal distension.
Spleen	Pain is the posterior mandibular region and lower cheek. Pain and coldness along the inside of the thigh and knee. Oedema of the legs and feet. Muscle wasting/weakness of the limbs. Digestive problems.
Heart	Pain in the scapular region and medial forearm. Pain in the back. Fullness and pain in the chest and lateral costal region. Hot/painful palms. Discomfort when lying flat. Dizziness and fainting.
Small Intestine	Pain on the lateral aspect of the shoulder and upper arm. Pain in the cheeks. Lower abdominal pain stretching around to the lumbar region. Back pain radiating into the testicles. Stomach pain with constipation. Dry mouth.
Bladder	Pain in the lumbar region, spine, posterior thigh, calf and foot. Stiff neck, headache, ocular pain, altered micturition.
Kidney	Backpain, pain in the lateral gluteal region, pain in the posterior aspect of the thigh, pain in the soles of the feet. Shortness of breath, restlessness, abdominal distension. Impotence.
Pericardium	Pain and stiffness in the neck. Limb spasm. Pain in the eyes. Subaxillary swelling. Fullness in the chest and lateral costal region. Palpitations.
Triple energizer	Pain on the posterior aspect of the shoulder and upper arm. Pain behind the ear. Tinnitus. Reddening and pain of the eyes. Abdominal distension.
Gallbladder	Pain in the lateral knee and fibula. Ocular pain. Headache. Pain under the chin. Pain in the lateral costal area and chest. Constant bitter taste in the mouth.
Liver	Spasm in the limbs. Headache. Tinnitus. Blurred vision. Lower abdominal pain.

(Adapted from Ellis et al., 1994)

Proportional measurement

Acupuncture points may be located in two ways. Firstly they may be placed in anatomical terms in relation to surface anatomy, using body landmarks. For example, the point HT-7 lies proximal to the pisiform bone on the radial side of flexor carpi ulnaris. Secondly, points may be located using proportional measurement. The unit of proportional measurement is the 'cun', and 1 cun is the width of the patient's thumb at the level of the interphalangeal joint. The breadth of the hand across all four fingers at the proximal interphalangeal joint is 3 cun, the width of the 2nd and 3rd fingers at this level is 1.5 cun. A number of proportional measurements are shown in Appendix 3.1.

Clinically the easiest method of measurement is to use the hand span (of the patient) or the thumb. In addition, measuring from the lateral joint line of the knee to the apex of the lateral malleolus is 16 cun. If this distance is measured in centimetres with a tape the distance is simply divided by 16 to find the single cun measurement for this particular patient. This should be recorded on the notes for future reference. For example, if the patient's tibial length measured as above is 42 cm, one cun is 42 divided by 16 which is 2.63 cm. For a point such as ST-36 which lies 3 cun below the knee joint line, the distance for this patient would be 3 times 2.63 which is 7.9 cm.

The 12 regular Meridians

Lung (LU)

The lung channel (Fig. 3.3) is said to begin internally near the stomach, in an area known as the middle jiao. From here, it travels downwards to connect with the large intestine and then returns to pass through the diaphragm and then into the lungs. The internal meridian ascends into the throat and then emerges at LU-1 in the first intercostal space 6 cun lateral to the midline. The external channel then travels upwards to LU-2 at the delto-pectoral triangle. From here the lung meridian travels along the antero-lateral aspect of the upper arm, lateral to the heart and pericardium meridians, to the cubital fossa at LU-5, at the radial side of the biceps tendon. The meridian travels on the lateral palmar aspect of the forearm towards the styloid process of the radius to LU-9 between the radial artery and the abductor pollicis longus tendon, level with the proximal border of the pisiform bone. Finally, the meridian moves across the thenar eminence to the radial nail point of the thumb at LU-11.

The lung luo-connecting channel separates from the primary channel at LU-7 to spread across the thenar eminence and connect with the large intestine channel. The lung divergent channel separates from the primary channel at the axilla and passes to the heart channel and the large intestine channel.

The lung channel is therefore connected (internally-externally paired) with the large intestine channel and its divergent channel ascends to the throat, hence sore throat and voice changes are often seen in lung conditions. The lung channel does not connect directly to the nose, but does so via the large intestine meridian, hence it is said that the lung 'opens to the nose' and the lung channel can be used to treat nasal disorders.

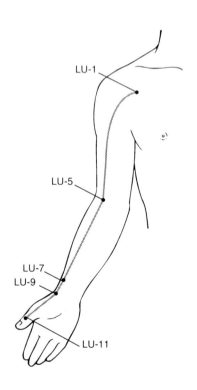

Figure 3.3. *Lung channel*

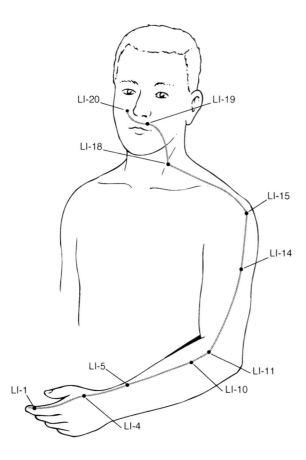

Figure 3.4. *Large intestine channel*

Large intestine (LI)

The large intestine channel (Fig. 3.4) begins at the radial side of the tip of the index finger and runs between the 1st and 2nd metacarpals to LI-4 (midpoint of the 2nd metacarpal bone close to its radial border), and then between the tendons of extensor pollicis longus and extensor pollicis brevis to enter the anatomical snuffbox at LI-5. It continues along the lateral aspect of the forearm to LI-11 at the elbow crease, approximately midway between the biceps tendon and the lateral epicondyle of the humerus. The channel travels up the lateral aspect of the upper arm to LI-15 anterior and inferior to the acromion process. From here it passes posteriorly to LI-16 between the lateral aspect of the clavicle and the scapular spine and then medially to the suprascapular fossa to GV-14 at the level of the seventh cervical vertebra where it meets the other five yang channels. At this point a branch of the channel travels internally to connect with the lung and travel down to the large intestine as far as ST-37 (3 cun inferior to ST-36) the lower he-sea point of the large intestine. The external meridian continues from the supraclavicular fossa to the lateral aspect of the neck, LI-18 lying between the two heads of sternomastoid level with the tip of the Adams apple. The meridian passes through the cheek to the lower gums. The channel crosses to the opposite side along the upper lip to terminate at the side of the nose at LI-20, where the large intestine

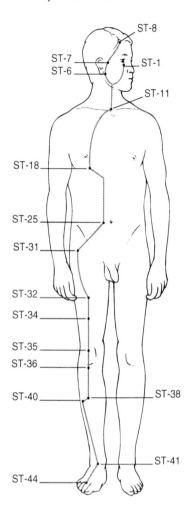

Figure 3.5. *Stomach channel*

channel joins the stomach channel.

The large intestine luo-connecting channel separates from the main meridian at LI-6 (3 cun proximal to LI-5, which lies in the centre of the anatomical snuffbox). It joins the lung channel and ascends to the shoulder, neck, and jaw where it divides giving one branch which travels forward to the teeth and a second which travels backwards to the ear. The large intestine divergent channel ascends the arm to LI-15 and then travels medially to the spine and back to the supraclavicular fossa. From here it also divides into two branches, one descending to the lung and large intestine and the other ascending to join the primary channel at the throat.

Stomach (ST)

The stomach channel (Fig. 3.5) begins internally at the lateral side of the nose at LI-20 and ascends to the medial canthus where it meets with the bladder channel at BL-1. The channel then travels laterally along the infra-orbital ridge to become external at ST-1. The channel descends and curves inwards to join the GV channel at GV-26 and then circles around the lips to meet the conception vessel at CV-24 in the groove of the chin. The meridian then runs laterally across the cheek to ST-6 at the angle of the jaw, and ascends to the ear (ST-7 lying anterior to the condyloid process) and hairline (ST-8 at the corner of the forehead). One branch of the channel separates at ST-5 and descends along the anterior border of the sternomastoid muscle to ST-12 in the supraclavicular fossa above the midline of the clavicle. An internal channel travels posteriorly and descends internally to connect with the stomach and spleen organs. The primary stomach channel descends along the mamillary line (4 cun lateral to the midline) to ST-18 (directly below the nipple in the 5th intercostal space) and then moves inwards to descend 2 cun lateral to the midline to ST-30 level with the superior border of the pubic symphasis. At this point the internal channel descends from the stomach organ to rejoin the main channel. The channel swings laterally to ST-31 over the neck of the femur and then descends over the antero-lateral aspect of the thigh and lateral aspect of the tibia to the dorsum of the foot, terminating at ST-45 on the lateral nail point of the second toe. A further branch separates from the main channel at ST-36 to descend internally to the lateral aspect of the third toe, and a final branch separates from the main channel at ST-42 to pass to the tip of the big toe to join the spleen channel at SP-1.

The stomach luo-connecting channel begins at ST-40, joins with the spleen channel and ascends to converge with the other yang channels in the neck. The stomach divergent channel separates from the main channel in the thigh and passes upwards to enter the abdomen, passing through the stomach, spleen and heart, and then emerges at the mouth.

Spleen (SP)

The spleen channel (Fig. 3.6) begins at the medial nail point of the 1st toe at SP-1, and runs along the medial aspect of the foot (between the light and dark skin) to begin its ascent at SP-5 (level with the anterior and inferior borders of the medial malleolus). The channel follows the posterior border of the tibia and then crosses the liver channel 8 cun superior to the medial malleolus. The channel ascends across the medial aspect of the knee and thigh to the lower abdomen where a branch travels internally to enter the spleen and stomach organs. The main channel ascends 4 cun lateral to the midline to SP-16 (level with CV-11, 3 cun above the umbilicus) where the channel moves out to 6 cun lateral to the midline at SP-17 (in the 5th intercostal space). The main channel travels upwards as far as LU-1 (1st intercostal space) and then descends to SP-21 in the 7th intercostal space on the mid-axillary line. Branches from the main channel run internally to the lower surface of the tongue and to the heart.

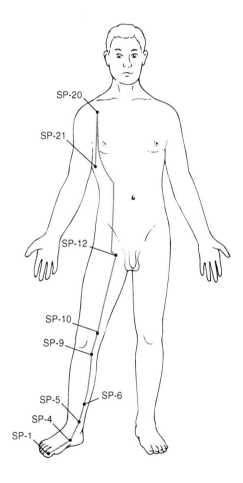

Figure 3.6. *Spleen channel*

The spleen luo-connecting channel originates at SP-4 (distal to the base of the 1st metatarsal bone) and links to the stomach channel to connect with the stomach and intestines. The spleen divergent channel branches from the main channel in the mid-thigh and joins the divergent channel of the stomach to ascend to the throat and tongue.

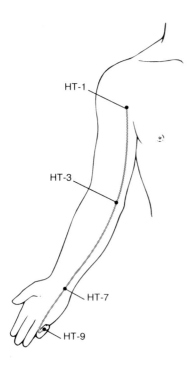

Figure 3.7. *Heart channel*

Heart (HT)

The heart channel (Fig. 3.7) begins in the heart organ and descends through the diaphragm to connect with the small intestine. A branch separates from the main channel and ascends with the oesophagus to the face to end in the tissues around the eye. The main meridian channel travels from the heart to the lung organ and emerges at HT-1 in the centre of the axilla. The channel travels along the medial aspect of the upper arm to HT-3 on the medial side of the elbow crease mid-way between the biceps tendon and the medial epicondyle of the humerus. The channel continues along the antero-medial side of the forearm to HT-7 at the wrist joint on the proximal border of the pisiform bone. From the wrist the channel travels through the palm and along the radial side of the 5th metacarpal and phalanx to the radial nail point of the 5th phalanx at HT-9. The heart luo-connecting channel separates from the main channel at HT-5 (1 cun proximal to HT-7) and connects with the small intestine channel to continue to the root of the tongue and the eye. The heart divergent channel separates from the primary channel at the axilla, descends to the heart and ascends to the throat and face again connecting with the small intestine channel at the inner canthus.

Small intestine (SI)

The small intestine channel (Fig. 3.8) begins at the ulnar nail point of the 5th finger (SI-1) and travels along the ulnar side of the 5th finger to the wrist at SI-4 (between the base of the 5th metacarpal and the triquetral bone). The channel ascends the forearm on the ulnar aspect to SI-8 (between the tip of the olecranon and the medial epicondyle of the humerus, directly over the ulnar nerve). The channel continues upwards on the posterior aspect of the upper arm crossing the large intestine meridian at LI-14 (insertion of the deltoid muscle) to the posterior aspect of the shoulder at SI-9 (1 cun superior to the posterior axillary crease) and SI-10 (in the depression below the scapular spine over the posterior aspect of the gleno-humeral joint). The channel forms a zigzag across the scapula and travels medially to SI-15 (2 cun lateral to C7). The channel travels up the neck in association with the sternomastoid muscle to SI-17 (between the angle of the mandible and the sternomastoid). The channel then crosses the cheek to SI-18 (directly below the outer canthus on the lower border of the zygomatic bone), and then swings posteriorly to SI-19 (over the tempero-mandibular joint). A branch from the primary channel travels to the outer canthus to meet the gallbladder meridian.

The small intestine luo-connecting channel leaves the primary channel at SI-7 (in the groove on the anterior border of the ulna 5 cun from the wrist joint) to connect with the heart channel. The small intestine divergent channel separates from the primary channel at the shoulder and descends to the small intestine organ.

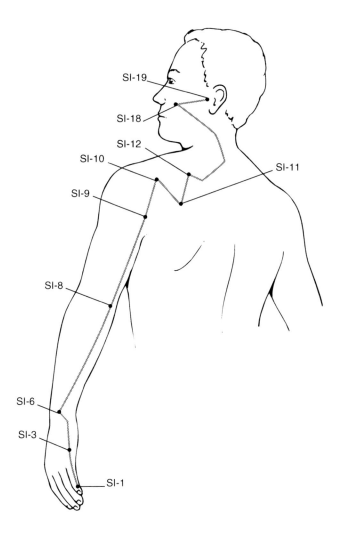

Figure 3.8. *Small intestine channel*

Bladder (BL)

The bladder channel begins (Fig. 3.9) at BL-1 on the inner canthus and ascends to the forehead and head. A branch descends to the temple and ear intersecting with the gallbladder channel. The primary channel travels over the back of the head to BL-9 (1.5 cun superior to the external occipital protuberance) and BL-10 over the transverse process of C1. The channel splits into inner and outer branches at this point.

The inner branch (from BL-11, level with T1) travels the length of the spine 1.5 lateral to the spinous processes. The inner branch descends as far as BL-30 (1.5 cun from the midline level with the 4th posterior sacral foramen). The channel then moves up again to BL-31 (over the 1st posterior sacral foramen) and then descends via the sacrum with each point over the respective sacral foramina (BL-32, 2nd. BL-33, 3rd. BL-34, 4th.) The channel then moves inwards to BL-35 0.5 cun from the tip of the coccyx and continues down to BL-36 at the buttock crease and then to BL-40 in the popliteal fossa.

The outer bladder line, beginning at BL-41 (level with T2) lies 3 cun

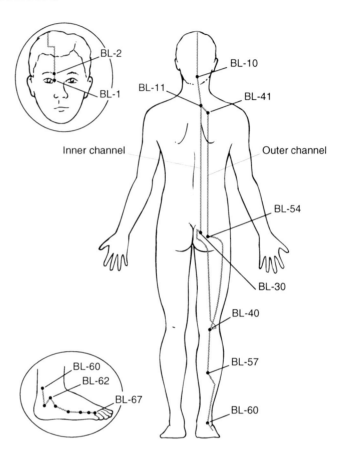

Figure 3.9. *Bladder channel*

lateral to the spinous processes. The outer branch continues as far as BL-54 (3 cun lateral to the sacral hiatus). It then crosses the buttock (intersecting with GB-30), and descends to re-join the inner channel in the popliteal fossa, BL-55 lying 2 cun inferior to BL-40 (centre of the popliteal fossa). The bladder channel continues to BL-57 (between the medial and lateral bellies of gastrocnemius) and BL-58 (1 cun lateral and inferior to BL-57). The channel passes down the back of the calf to the outside of the ankle at BL-60 (between the lateral malleolus and the Achilles), and then to the calcaneum at BL-61 (midway between BL-60 and the skin covering the heel) and then upwards to BL-62 (inferior to the lateral malleolus just posterior to the peroneal tendons). The channel continues along the outer edge of the foot to the fifth metatarsal to terminate at the lateral nail point of the 5th toe at BL-67.

The bladder luo-connecting channel separates at BL-58 to join with the kidney channel. The bladder divergent channel leaves the primary channel in the popliteal fossa (BL-40) and ascends to the sacrum and anus and connects with the bladder and kidney organs.

Kidney (KI)

The kidney meridian (Fig. 3.10) begins on the sole of the foot at KI-1. It passes medially to KI-2 anterior and inferior to the tuberosity of navicular, and then passes behind the medial malleolus to KI-3 (midway between the medial malleolus and the Achilles tendon). The meridian forms a loop, dropping down to KI-5 (1 cun inferior to KI-3) and then up again to KI-6 (1 cun below the prominence of the medial malleolus). The meridian ascends along the medial aspect of the leg intersecting with the spleen and liver meridians at SP-6 (the 'three yin intersection', or '*Sanyinjiao*'). The primary meridian continues to the medial aspect of the popliteal crease at KI-10 (between the tendons of semimembranosus and semitendinosus), and then ascends along the postero-medial aspect of the thigh to the tip of the coccyx. From here a branch of the meridian passes internally to the spine and enters the kidney organ and connects to the bladder. One branch passes up through the liver and lung to terminate at the root of the tongue. Another branch joins the heart and links to the pericardium channel at CV-17 (front mu point of the pericardium channel). At this point the kidney, small intestine, spleen and Triple Energiser channels meet with the CV (conception) channel. The primary channel continues to KI-11 at the superior border of the symphasis pubis 0.5 cun lateral to the midline. The channel ascends 0.5 cun from the midline to KI-21 (level with CV-14, 6 cun above the umbilicus) where the channel moves laterally to KI-22 (in the 5th intercostal space) and now ascends 2 cun lateral to the midline, to terminate at KI-27 in the depression on the lower border of the clavicle.

The kidney divergent channel separates from the primary channel in the popliteal fossa and ascends through the lumbar spine to the kidney organ and on to the neck and root of the tongue. This pathway is important in relation to the main use of the channel in musculoskeletal therapy, that is, treatment of chronic low back pain.

The kidney luo-connecting channel begins at KI-4 and connects with the bladder.

Pericardium

The pericardium channel (Fig. 3.11) originates in the centre of the chest. One branch travels internally down through the diaphragm to the abdomen (lower jiao). The other branch travels across the chest to emerge at PC-1 (1 cun lateral to the nipple in the 4th intercostal space). The meridian passes over the axilla to travel down the antero-medial aspect of the arm between the lung and heart channels to reach the elbow at PC-3 (on the elbow crease, at the ulnar side of the biceps tendon). The primary channel descends down the forearm between palmaris longus and flexor carpi radialis to PC-7 lying between the tendons of these two muscles at the wrist crease. The channel passes into the hand to PC-8 between the 2nd and 3rd metacarpals (at the tip of the middle finger when a loose fist is formed) to terminate at PC-9 at the radial nail point of the middle finger.

The pericardium luo-connecting channel begins at PC-6 (2 cun proximal to PC-7 at the wrist crease) and joins with the heart channel. The pericardium divergent channel separates from the primary channel inferior to the axilla to enter the chest. Another branch ascends to the throat and emerges behind the ear to join the Triple Energiser channel.

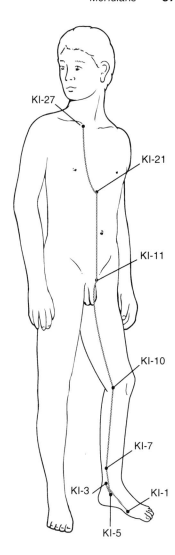

Figure 3.10. *Kidney channel*

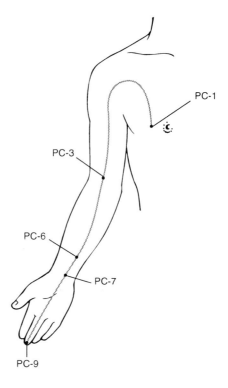

Figure 3.11. *Pericardium channel*

Triple Energiser (TE)

The Triple Energiser channel or 'Sanjiao' (Fig. 3.12) begins on the ulnar side of the 4th (ring) finger and travels between the 3rd and 4th fingers (TE-2 and TE-3) to the wrist, TE-4 lying between the tendons of extensor digiti minimi and extensor digitorum communis at the wrist crease. From here the channel travels between the radius and ulna along the posterior aspect of the forearm to TE-10 1 cun proximal to the tip of the olecranon. The meridian runs along the lateral aspect of the upper arm to TE-14 in the depression posterior to the acromion. The meridian intersects with the gallbladder meridian and then descends to the supraclavicular fossa, TE-15 lying 1 cun posterior to GB-21. The main meridian passes upwards to the posterior border of sternomastoid (TE-16) and then to the bottom of the ear, TE-17 lying between the ramus of the mandible and the mastoid process. The meridian winds around the ear to TE-20 on the side of the head at the apex of the auricle, and down to TE-21 superior to the condyloid process of the mandible. From here the meridian passes forwards along the temple (TE-22) to the lateral end of the eyebrow at TE-23.

The divergent channel separates from the main channel on the side of the head, one branch passing upwards to the vertex of the head, the other downwards to the chest and abdomen. The Triple Energiser luo-connecting channel separates from the main channel at TE-5 to connect with the pericardium meridian.

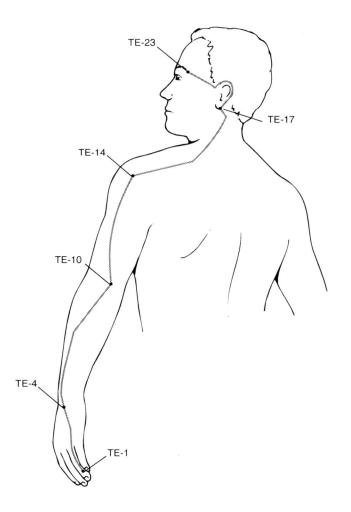

Figure 3.12. *Triple Energiser (Sanjiao) channel*

Gallbladder (GB)

The gallbladder channel (Fig. 3.13) starts on the outer canthus of the eye (GB-1) and crosses to the condyloid process in front of the ear (GB-2). From here the meridian moves upwards and forwards to the temporal region, just within the hairline (GB-4), and then down again to meet with the Triple Energiser meridian, GB-7 lying one fingerbreadth anterior to TE-20 at the apex of the auricle. The meridian curves around the ear and descends to GB-12 in the depression posterior and inferior to the mastoid process. The meridian curves upwards once again on the side of the head and travels over the forehead to GB-14 lying 1 cun above the centre of the eyebrow. Once again the meridian changes direction to curve over the side of the head and down to the apex of the neck at GB-20 lying midway between the origins of the sternomastoid and trapezius muscles. From here the gallbladder meridian travels to the shoulder lying at the crest of the upper trapezius (GB-21) and then downwards and outwards along the side of the chest to GB-22 and GB-23 in the 5th intercostal space. The meridian moves inwards to GB-24 lying below the nipple in the 7th

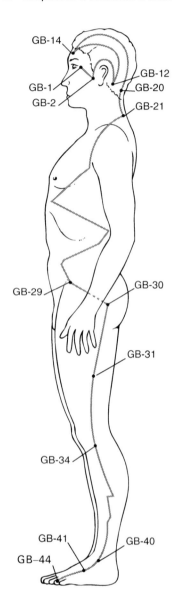

Figure 3.13. *Gallbladder channel*

intercostal space. It then swings outwards to GB-25 at the free end of the 12th rib, and circles forwards and downwards to the postero-lateral aspect of the hip joint at GB-30. The meridian then descends along the lateral aspect of the leg (ilio-tibial band) to pass in front of the head of the fibula (GB-34) and in front of the lateral malleolus (GB-40) to end at the lateral nail point of the 4th toe (GB-44).

A minor branch from the primary channel enters the ear, while another meets with the Triple Energiser meridian. This latter branch descends to the neck to meet the primary channel again in the suprascapular fossa. Another branch from the primary meridian separates in the supraclavicular region to descend internally through the diaphragm to connect with the liver and then enter the gallbladder. The internal branch meets with the primary channel again in the hip region. A further branch leaves the primary channel at GB-41 to enter the 1st toe.

The gallbladder luo-connecting channel leaves the primary channel at GB-37 (5 cun superior to the apex of the lateral malleolus on the anterior border of the fibula) to connect with the liver channel. The gallbladder divergent channel leaves the primary channel in the thigh to enter the pubic hairline and merge with the divergent channel of the liver. This channel travels upwards across the heart and oesophagus to the face to rejoin the primary channel at the outer canthus.

Liver (LR)

The liver meridian (Fig 3.14) originates on the lateral nail point of the 1st toe (LR-1) and travels along the dorsum of the foot between the 1st and 2nd toes. The meridian passes to the medial aspect of the ankle, LR-4 lying anterior to the prominence of the medial malleolus. It intersects with the spleen channel at SP-6 (3 cun superior to the apex of the medial malleolus) and rises to a point 8 cun above the malleolus where it crosses behind the spleen channel to continue to the knee, (LR-8 lying just superior to the medial edge of the popliteal crease) and thigh (LR-12 lying medial to the femoral vein in the crease of the groin). The meridian continues to the pubic region where it curves around the genitalia to the abdomen. It ascends to the free end of the 11th rib (LR-13) and then to the 6th intercostal space on the mamillary line (LR-14).

A branch from the primary channel enters the abdomen to curve around the stomach, connect with the gallbladder and enters the liver. This branch spreads to the lung and upwards through the neck and throat to the nasopharynx to connect with the eye tissues. The branch then emerges from the forehead to merge with the governor vessel at the vertex of the head (GV-20).

The liver luo-connecting channel separates from the primary channel at LR-5 to connect with the gallbladder channel. The liver divergent channel separates from the primary channel on the dorsum of the foot to ascend to the pubic region and join with the gallbladder primary channel.

Conception vessel (CV)

The conception (CV) vessel (Fig. 3.15) begins at CV-1 in the perineum, between the anus and external genitalia, and ascends along the midline

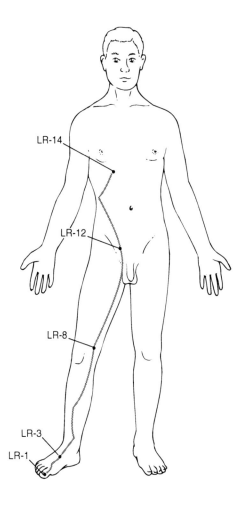

Figure 3.14. *Liver channel*

of the body. The meridian passes across the centre of the pubic symphasis (CV-2) and the umbilicus (CV-8) and rises to the sternocostal angle (CV-16) midpoint of the nipple line (CV-17) and jugular notch (CV-22). The conception vessel terminates above the chin in the depression central to the mentolabial groove (CV-24).

The interior portion of the channel connects with the governing vessel at GV-28 and connects with the stomach channel at ST-1. A branch from the conception vessel passes from the pelvic cavity to ascend along the spine. The conception luo-connecting vessel passes from CV-15 into the abdomen.

Governing vessel (GV)

The governing vessel (GV) (Fig. 3.16) begins at GV-1 in the perineum between the coccyx and the anus. The vessel passes posteriorly along the interior of the spinal column, GV-2 at the sacro-coccygeal hiatus, GV-4 at the lower border of the L2 spinous process. GV-6 below the spinous process of T11, and GV-14 below the spinous process of C7. GV-16 lies below the external occipital protuberance and from here the

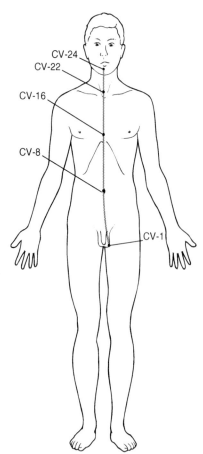

Figure 3.15. *Conception (CV) channel*

vessel arches over the back of the head to GV-20 at the vertex of the head. From GV-16 a branch enters the brain. The vessel continues to arch over the forehead and along the centre of the nose to GV-26 above the upper lip (the philtrum).

The eight extra channels

In addition to the 12 regular meridians, eight extra (extraordinary) channels also exist. The extra channels are closely associated to the function of the kidneys in Chinese medicine (Ross, 1998). The extra channels act as an 'overflow system' for qi (vital energy), jing (essence), and blood. In excess conditions, qi can be transferred from the regular meridians into the extra channels, and in cases of deficiency the extra channels can 'top up' the regular channels acting as a reserve of energy.

The extra vessels also link the 12 regular channels. The **Governor Vessel** links all six yang channels at GV-14 ('sea of yang' or 'sea of qi') while the **Conception Vessel** links all the yin channels. The **penetrating vessel** links the stomach and kidney channels and strengthens the link between the conception and governing channels. It is known as the 'sea of the twelve primary channels' or the 'sea of blood' (Deadman et al., 1998). The **girdle vessel** encircles the abdomen and binds the vertical paths of the primary channels. The **yin motility vessel** is said to dominate quietness while the **yang motility vessel** is said to dominate activity. The **yin linking vessel** dominates the interior of the whole body and the **yang linking vessel** dominates the exterior of the whole body.

The term 'mai' means vessels and so the eight extraordinary meridians are termed 'mai' (Table 3.3). The governing vessel (Du mai) and conception vessel (Ren mai) run along the back and front of the body. The penetrating vessel (Chong mai) travels up the centre of the body from the abdomen to the chest, ascending via the kidney channel (KI-11 to KI-21). The girdle vessel (Dai mai) circles the trunk at the level of LR-13 and travels with the gallbladder channel (GB-26 to GB-28). The word 'qiao' means heel and so the next two meridians are termed heel or motility vessels. The qiao mai vessels start below the malleoli, the yang motility vessel (yang qiao mai) beginning below the lateral malleolus while the yin motility vessel (yin qiao mai) begins below the medial malleolus. The word 'wei' means connection or network, hence the descriptive term 'linking vessel'. The yang linking vessel (yang wei mai) connects the exterior (yang) of the body and travels on the outside of the leg and ascends through the back to connect with the governing channel. The yin linking vessel (yin wei mai) connects the interior (yin) of the body and travels over the front of the body connecting with the conception channel.

The extra channels differ from the regular meridians in that they are not directly related to the individual Zang Fu organs. In addition, only the GV and CV channels possess their own points, the other six of the extra channels borrow points from the regular meridians. The GV and CV channels are described above, the other extra meridians are shown in Table 3.4.

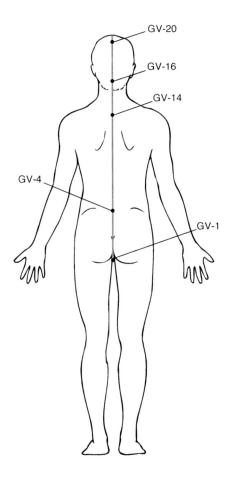

Figure 3.16. *Governing (GV) channel*

Table 3.3. The eight extra (extraordinary) meridians.

Chinese name	English equivalent
Du mai	Governing channel
Ren mai	Conception channel
Chong mai	Penetrating channel
Dai mai	Girdle channel
Yang qiao mai	Yang heel (motility) channel
Yin qiao mai	Yin heel (motility) channel
Yin wei mai	Yin linking channel
Yang wei mai	Yang linking channel

The extra vessels may be activated and brought into a treatment by using the eight confluence points all of which lie above the wrist or below the ankle (Table 3.5) and are described on page 68.

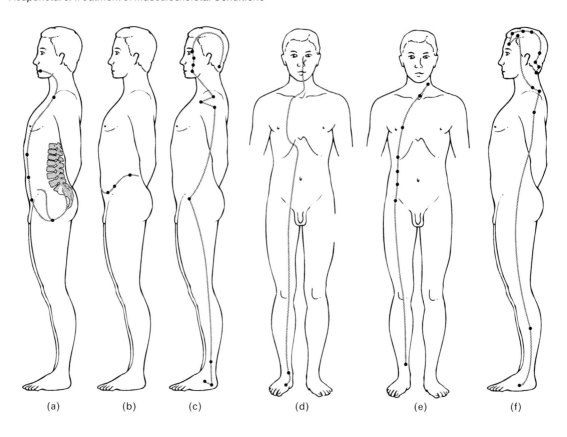

(a)   (b)   (c)   (d)   (e)   (f)

Table 3.4. The extra meridians.

(a) *Penetrating vessel*
Originates in the lower abdomen to emerge at CV-1. Ascends in the spine to emerge near ST-30 to connect with the kidney meridian, running with it from KI-11 to KI-21. Travels to the throat and lips.

(b) *Girdle vessel*
Begins near LR-13 and runs around the waist through GB-26, GB-27 and GB-28.

(c) *Yang motility vessel*
Begins at the lateral malleolus (BL-62) and runs posterior to the fibula and along the lateral aspect of the thigh. Travels along the posterior aspect of the chest to pass behind the axilla and wind around the shoulder. Ascends along the neck to the corner of the mouth and inner canthus (BL-1) to meet with the yin motility vessel.

(d) *Yin motility vessel*
Begins at the medial malleolus (KI-6) and runs upwards along the medial aspect of the thigh to the groin and then along the chest to the suprascapular fossa. Passes to the throat to reach BL-1 at the inner canthus and merge with the yang motility vessel.

(e) *Yang linking vessel*
Starts from the heel (BL-63) to pass to the lateral malleolus and ascend along the gallbladder meridian. Passes through the hip region and along the posterior chest to the shoulder and then to the forehead. Travels back to the posterior aspect of the neck to enter GV-15 and GV-16.

(f) *Yin linking vessel*
Begins on the medial aspect of the leg at KI-9 and ascends along the medial aspect of the thigh and abdomen to communicate with the spleen meridian. Travels medially across the chest to link with the conception vessel at CV-22 and CV-23.

Table 3.5. Activating the eight extra meridians using the confluence points.

Extra meridian	Confluence points	Indications	Main functions
Penetrating/Yin linking	SP-4/PC-6	Heart and circulatory disorders. Gastrointestinal (GI) disorders. Blood stasis, gynaecological conditions. Fullness of the chest.	Circulates energy throughout internal organs Links heart and digestive functions. Prevents blood stasis. Regulates the physical and spiritual heart.
Girdling/Yang linking	GB-41/TE-5	Symptoms of the lateral side of the body. Weakness of the abdomen and low back.	Binds the exterior and braces the back and lower abdomen. Causes yang to descend.
Du/Yang motility	SI-3/BL-62	Symptoms of the head, neck and back. Central nervous system (CNS) disorders.	Stores yang and causes it to ascend to head and eyes. Distributes yang. Especially useful when treating illness in males.
Ren/Yin motility	LU-7/KI-6	Disorders of the throat and lungs. Gynaecological and urinary disorders. Conditions affecting the abdominal organs.	Stores yin and causes it to ascend and nourish head and eyes. Distributes yin in general. Especially useful when treating illness in females.

(Pirog, 1996; Xinnong, 1999)

Appendix 3.1

Cun measurements

The distance between the nipples is 8 cun.
The distance between the mid-point of the clavicles is 8 cun.
The distance between the tip of the acromium process and the midline of the body is 8 cun.
The distance between the anterior axillary and cubital creases is 12 cun.
The distance between the cubital creases and the wrist creases is 12 cun.
The distance between the sternocostal angle and the umbilicus is 8 cun.

The distance between the mastoid processes is 9 cun.
The distance between the posterior hairline and the inferior border of the spinous process of C7 is 3 cun.
The distance between the medial borders of the scapulae is 6 cun.

The distance between the ends of the creases of the interphalangeal joints of the middle finger at their widest point is 1 cun.
The distance between the proximal phalangeal joint and the tip of the index finger is 2 cun.
The width of the interphalangeal joint of the thumb is 1 cun.

The width of the four fingers, held close together at the level of the dorsal skin crease of the proximal interphalangeal joint of the middle finger, is 3 cun.

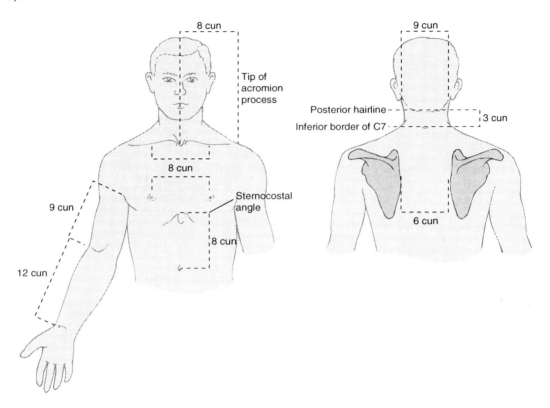

The width of the index and middle fingers, held close together at the level of the dorsal skin crease of the proximal interphalangeal joint of the middle finger, is 1.5 cun.

The distance between the angles of the hairline is 9 cun.

The distance between the anterior and posterior hairlines is 12 cun.
The distance between the glabella and the anterior hairline is 3 cun.

The distance between the umbilicus and the pubic symphysis is 5 cun.
The distance between the lateral prominence of the greater trochanter (approximately level with the inferior border of the pubic symphysis) and the popliteal crease is 19 cun.
The height of the patella is 2 cun.
The distance between the gluteal fold and the knee is 14 cun.
The distance between the popliteal crease and the lateral malleolus is 16 cun.
The distance between the popliteal crease and the medial malleolus is 15 cun.

(Reproduced with permission from Deadman et al., 1998)

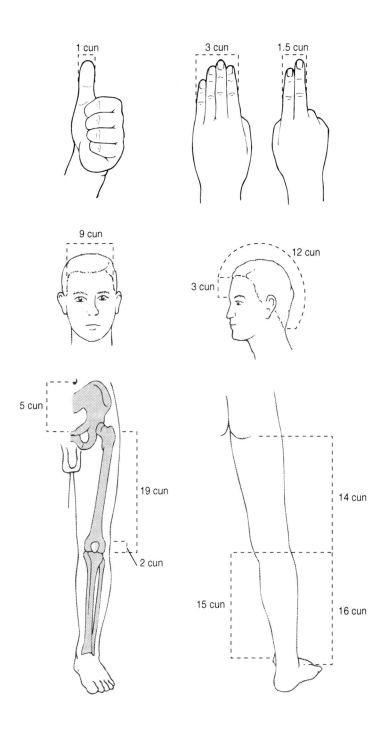

Acupuncture and pain relief

Neurophysiological concepts of pain

Pain may be defined as a sensation resulting from a stimulus which is intense enough to threaten to cause injury (Bray, 1986). The stimulus itself may be thermal, mechanical or chemical in nature and often a combination of these. Receptors in the body which register pain are called nociceptors (pain receptors) and are supplied by either small myelinated $A\delta$ fibres or unmyelinated C fibres. $A\delta$ fibres only signal high intensity stimuli while the C fibres signal a broader array of stimuli including high intensity, chemical and thermal stimuli. Being myelinated, the $A\delta$ fibres are responsible for 'fast' pain and give rise to the initial feeling of well-localised pain. They often trigger a flexor withdrawal reflex helping the body to avoid potential harm. C fibres give rise to 'slow' pain, which creates a dull aching, throbbing sensation and is poorly defined and longer lasting. Often both fibres will respond to intense stimuli giving a well-defined ($A\delta$) sharp sensation followed by a dull, aching (C) after shadow. While fast pain gives the opportunity for avoidance, slow pain is thought to enforce inactivity and is often associated with muscle spasm.

A number of fibres have been shown to be involved during acupuncture pain relief, and give various sensations on needling, but it is the $A\delta$ and C fibres which have the greatest involvement in acupuncture pain relief.

The small unmyelinated C fibres represent the most common of the afferent nerves seen in mammals. They receive impulses from free nerve endings in the skin and deep tissues, and travel to the spinal cord to give off branches travelling upwards and downwards for a number of spinal segments (Fig. 4.1). The branches terminate in the dorsal horn of the spinal cord making contact with the substantia gelatinosa (SG) cells in lamina II in the gray matter of the cord. From lamina II, the impulses converge on wide dynamic range (WDR) cells in lamina V (Fig. 4.2).

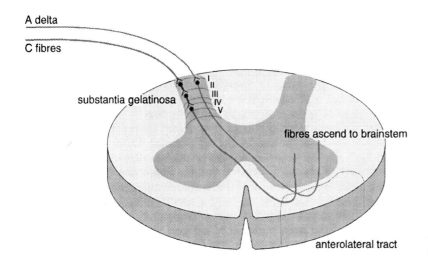

Figure 4.1. *Segment of spinal cord showing C and Aδ fibre routes. (Reproduced with permission from White, 1999)*

The impulses from the SG travel in the spinoreticular tract on the opposite side of the spinal cord to the reticular formation of the brain. The reticular formation can be considered as the arousal system of the brain and is thought to play a large part in integrating feelings of pain with its behavioural response (White, 1999). From here, the nociceptive stimuli pass to the thalamus and then to the cerebral cortex. Some of the fibres travel to the limbic system, especially the cingulate gyrus, to create an emotional impact. C fibres thus give pain which although poorly localised has considerable emotional affect (White, 1999).

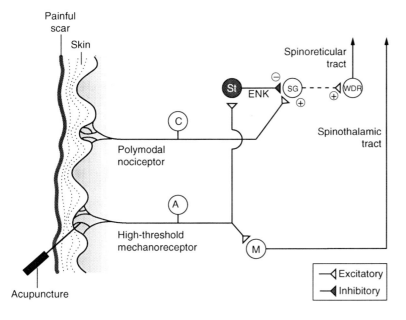

Figure 4.2. *C fibre connection to wide dynamic range (WDR) cells*

The C fibres use two amino acids as transmitters, glutamate and aspartate. In acute pain, the release of glutamate stimulates the release of AMPA (α-amino-3-hydroxy-5-methyl-4-isoxalone propionic acid) whereas in chronic pain glutamine leads to peptide release, which activates a second receptor, greatly amplifying (by up to 20 times) the original signal, a phenomenon known as 'central hypersensitivity'.

Aδ ('pinprick') fibres again travel to lamina II and V where they synapse with marginal cells and then travel to the brainstem via the spinothalamic tract running to the ventrobasal nuclei of the thalamus. From here, further neurons project to the sensory cortex.

In the SG of the cord some of the Aα fibres also synapse with the stalked cells (Bowsher, 1998) which release enkephalin to inhibit the SG and therefore block the pain impulses travelling into the SG via the C fibres. The stalked cells fire most effectively at 3Hz (Bowsher, 1998) and it is this frequency which is often used for electroacupuncture.

The Aα fibres provide rapid (myelinated) perception which is well localised. The Aα fibres travel to the reticular formation and thalamus and from here to the arcuate nucleus of the hypothalamus. This is the beginning of the descending inhibition system.

Descending inhibition activates a chain of neurons throughout the spinal cord. Two separate systems are involved, one involving serotonin, the other noradrenaline (Fig. 4.3). In the first system, fibres from the peri-aqueductal gray matter travel to the nucleus raphe magnus and then down the spinal cord to the stalked cells in the dorsal horn of the cord. Serotonin is released by the descending nerve fibres to activate the stalked cells leading to the release of enkephalin which in turn inhibits the SG cells. In the second system the arcuate nucleus of the hypothalamus activates nuclei in the brainstem. Descending fibres then release noradrenaline into the dorsal horn of the spinal cord to directly inhibit the SG cells.

These pathways are all used during acupuncture treatment. When the skin and underlying tissue is needled, Aδ fibres are stimulated via mechanoreceptors. The fibres travel to the brain to release opioids (mainly enkephalin) which inhibits transmission by C fibres. Aα fibres also travel to the cerebral cortex giving awareness of needling and causing the release of β endorphin. This substance in turn begins the process of descending inhibition involving serotonin. The descending neuron then causes pain inhibition by releasing opioids into the dorsal horn of the spinal cord. Four neurotransmitters have been found to be involved during acupuncture, serotonin (also called 5-hydroxytryptamine or 5-HT), β endorphin, enkephalin and dynorphins. It has been shown that electrical stimulation using electroacupuncture of low frequency (4 Hz) releases β endorphin, enkephalin and dynorphins. High frequency stimulation (200 Hz) releases dynorphins and serotonin. Prolonged stimulation may also release antagonists to these substances such as cholecystokinin and this may be the basis for the build up of acupuncture tolerance seen with repeated needling (White, 1999).

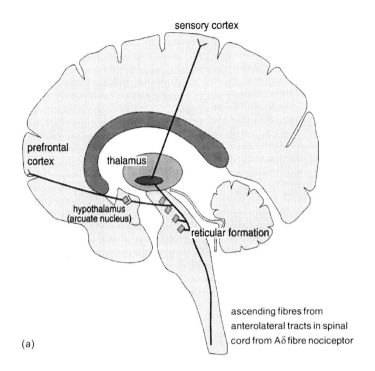

sensory cortex

prefrontal
cortex

thalamus

hypothalamus
(arcuate nucleus)

reticular formation

ascending fibres from
anterolateral tracts in spinal
cord from Aδ fibre nociceptor

(a)

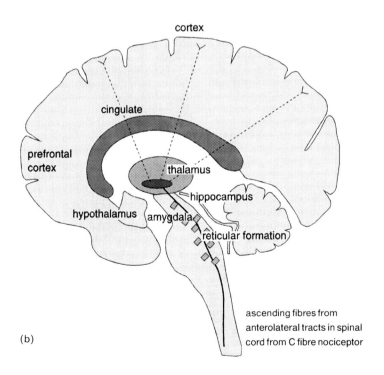

cortex

cingulate

prefrontal
cortex

thalamus

hippocampus

hypothalamus   amygdala

reticular formation

ascending fibres from
anterolateral tracts in spinal
cord from C fibre nociceptor

(b)

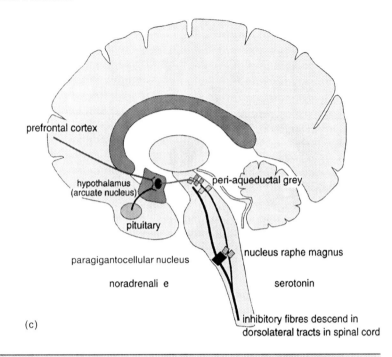

prefrontal cortex

hypothalamus
(arcuate nucleus)

peri-aqueductal grey

pituitary

paragigantocellular nucleus

nucleus raphe magnus

noradrenali e

serotonin

inhibitory fibres descend in
dorsolateral tracts in spinal cord

(c)

Figure 4.3. *(a–c) Pain pathways. (Reproduced with permission from White, 1999)*

Concepts of pain in traditional Chinese medicine

In TCM the flow of qi through the meridian system is central to the maintenance of health. When the flow is interrupted, health suffers, and pain may result.

Types of pain

We have seen in Chapter 1 that conditions may be described as *excess* or *deficient*, and similarly pain may also be described as excess or deficient. The terms full and empty may also be used (Maciocia, 1989). Excess-type pain occurs through an interruption in the free flow of qi within the meridian channels, and may be due to three main factors, *stagnation, obstruction* or through the influence of a *pathogen*. These three factors may occur individually or more usually in combination and in each case there is a build up of qi. Deficiency-type pain results from too little body fluids, qi, or yin. Pain in this case is caused by malnourishment of the channels.

Excess and deficiency pain differentiation

An excess pain occurs in the presence of a pathogenic factor (interior or exterior). The qi of the body remains intact and able to battle against the pathogen. If a pathogen attacks the body externally the flow of qi and blood through the meridians will slow and eventually stagnate. For example, pathogenic cold is said to cause contraction of the meridian channels which creates a ripple effect, and in turn causes pain. Warming the channel with the body's yang qi will cause the channel to relax and pain will be relieved (Ni, 1995).

Deficiency conditions usually occurs in the absence of a pathogen and are due to weakness of the body's qi. Typical signs on observation are used to differentiate excess/deficiency conditions and are shown in Table 4.1. On the whole deficiency conditions are chronic, with pain eased by pressure. These contrast with excess conditions which present as acute conditions where pain is aggravated by pressure.

Table 4.1. Differentiation between excess and deficiency conditions by patient observation.

Excess	Deficiency
Strong, load voice	Weak voice
Intense pain	Dull, lingering pain
Pain aggravated by pressure	Pain eased by pressure
Pain eased with movement	Pain eased with rest
Marked facial redness	Marked pale face
Profuse sweating	Slight sweating
Restlessness	Listlessness
Discards bedclothes at night	Curling up in bed
Outbursts of temper	Quiet disposition
Strong pulse	Weak pulse
Dry tongue with little coating	Thick/sticky tongue

Excess conditions include those exterior conditions due to invasion of exterior cold/wind/damp or heat (see Bi syndrome below). Interior conditions which are excess in nature include those of interior cold, heat, damp, wind, fire and phlegm, providing in each case the body's qi is strong enough to combat the pathogen. Stagnation of qi and or blood and also interior excess conditions.

Deficiency conditions can be further categorised into one of four types, deficiency of qi, yang, blood or yin. In addition to the signs shown in Table 4.1, these deficiency conditions may be differentiated by the presence of heat (deficiency of yin) or cold (deficiency of yang) in the limbs and by the organ affected. Deficiency of qi tends to affect the lung and spleen, deficiency of blood, the liver, heart and spleen. In each case further signs are shown dependent on the organ affected.

Stagnation may occur chiefly to qi or blood. Qi stagnation occurs when a body part or organ is obstructed or retarded, and qi can therefore no longer flow freely. The sensation is one of both pain and importantly distension, or a sense of 'fullness' or 'pressure'. Stagnation in musculoskeletal disorders may be due to soft tissue injury, but may also be due to factors such as improper diet, mental depression or pathogenic invasion. Initially qi circulation is hindered and finally totally obstructed, leading to a build up of qi behind the obstruction.

The feeling of distension is often worse than that of the pain itself, and the position of both distension and pain may change (Table 4.2).

Table 4.2. Nature of pain sensation.

Pain type	Indicating
Distending	Severe distension, but mild pain, moving from place to place. Indicates *qi stagnation.*
Pricking	Sharp and of fixed location, due to *stagnation of blood.*
Heaviness	Pain and heaviness show the presence of *damp*, blocking qi and/or blood.
Colicky	Sign of sudden *obstruction of qi* by substantial pathogen.
Pulling	Spasmodic in nature and of short duration. Caused by *wind* and usually related to the liver.
Burning	Burning together with a preference for cold. Due to invasion of collaterals by pathogenic *heat*, or excessive yang heat due to yin deficiency.
Cold	Together with a preference for warmth. Due to pathogenic *cold* blocking the collaterals or lack of warmth/nourishment of organs by qi.
Dull	Slight pain which lingers for long periods, showing *cold* syndrome of deficiency type.
Hollow	*Deficiency of blood* leading to emptiness of vessels.

The bi syndrome

Bi syndrome, also called 'painful obstruction syndrome' results in pain caused through *obstruction* of qi and blood due to *pathological invasion* of a combination of wind, cold and damp. Invasion is of all three pathogens, but one may take precedence over the other two. The condition is especially common in areas where the weather is cold, wet and windy and as such the bi syndrome is seen frequently in the UK and other northern European countries. The common factor is that pain is aggravated by the weather and may vary from mild joint discomfort, to severe disabling pain accompanied by swelling and joint deformity. The syndromes are traditionally classified into four classic types any of which may progress to a fifth (chronic) category (Table 4.3).

Table 4.3. Categories of bi syndrome.

Category	Character
Wandering	Pain moves from joint to joint, caused by pathogenic *wind.*
Painful	Severe pain caused by pathogenic *cold.*
Fixed	Soreness and heaviness caused by pathogenic *damp.*
Heat	Sudden onset with swelling and *redness.*
Bone (chronic)	Pain, swelling and joint *deformity.* Chronic (interior) condition, as a progression of the four previous types.

Wandering bi is seen especially in the peripheral limb joints including the wrist/elbows and knees/ankles. There may be chills and fever as a result of defensive qi fighting the pathogenic wind. The tongue coating may be thin and sticky and the pulse superficial reflecting an exterior syndrome. *Painful bi* presents as severe stabbing pains which are alleviated by heat (warmth) and aggravated by cold. The location is fixed in contrast to wandering bi and there is no local redness or heat (in contrast to heat bi). The excessive cold retards (slows) the flow of qi and blood but does not completely stop it. Cold is yin in character and tends to cause contraction while heat is yang and causes expansion (swelling). The contraction effect of the cold therefore dictates that the pain does not spread. Pain is alleviated by warmth because the warmth stimulates the flow of qi and blood to reduce the stagnation. Cold on the other hand makes the pain worse as it increases stagnation. The presence of pathogenic cold gives a white tongue coating and a string-tight pulse reflecting the association with cold and pain combined. *Fixed bi* is especially aggravated by cloudy and wet weather reflecting the invasion of damp as the main pathogen with this condition. Numbness and heaviness in the limbs is a sign of damp, and the tongue coating is white and sticky while the pulse is soft. Damp is a yin factor (as with cold) and so pain is localised to individual joints. *Heat bi* involves several joints and pain is severe, usually presenting with limitation of movement. There is swelling in the joints and there may be some deformity. The condition is associated with fever (without chills) and thirst, the tongue coating is yellow and the pulse rapid, both reflecting heat.

Bone bi or chronic painful obstructive syndrome is a progression of any of the four other types. Persistent attack by pathogens of the wind/cold/damp type lead to the development of phlegm, itself giving further obstruction. This greater obstruction gives muscular atrophy together with swelling and bony deformity. At this stage the bi syndrome moves from exterior to interior affecting the Zang Fu organs themselves. Prolonged attack by cold/wind/damp may lead to blood stasis, giving marked stiffness of the area. This progression shows the liver and kidneys to be affected and phlegm formation occurs. The liver functions to nourish the sinews and it is this functional decrement which leads to stiffness. The kidneys nourish bone and kidney deficiency causes the build up of phlegm in the joints causing swelling and deformity.

The essential aetiology of bi syndrome is a combination of attack by external pathogens (wind, cold and damp) upon a subject with a weakened body constitution. There is a temporary imbalance in the body such that the invasion of the pathogen is relatively stronger than the defence of the body to repel it. In the presence of a strong constitution the subject may not be affected, even though the pathogenic attack is marked. Equally, where the constitution is very weak, minimal pathogenic attack may be all that is required to cause bi syndrome. Importantly this is an external condition, the pathogen only affecting the channels. The individual only has a temporary and relative weakness of qi and blood, symptoms of prolonged qi or blood deficiency showing as internal effects. One of the essential factors is cold, wind and damp giving *stagnation* of blood and qi, and equally important is weakness of the body giving poor function of the pores which allows the invasion to take place.

Treatment is aimed at ahshi points, and distal points along the yang meridians travelling across the affected area. Wandering bi and heat bi are treated using the *reducing method* while fixed bi is treated using a *reinforcing method* with moxabustion and/or warm needling. Points are selected to eliminate all three pathogens, but emphasising the one single pathogen which dominates the condition (either wind, damp, or cold). Defensive qi and nutritive qi is reinforced, and deep insertion and needle retention is used where bone is affected. GB-20 is one of the most important points for eliminating wind, and blood may be nourished using BL-17 the meeting point of blood. Nourishing the blood will extinguish wind (Maciocia, 1994). SP-5 and SP-6 may both be used to eliminate dampness. SP-5 fortifies the spleen alone while SP-6 also harmonises the liver and kidney. In addition BL-20 may be used in cases of dampness as it is the back shu point of the Spleen. ST-36 also fortifies the spleen and removes dampness, but will additionally act to harmonise the stomach (internally connected to the spleen). GB-40 is the influential point of tendons and this may be used for classic bi syndromes. BL-11 is the influential point for bone, and GB-39 is the influential point for marrow, and both points may be chosen to treat bone bi syndrome. Both GV-14 and BL-23 may be used to tonify yang in cases of cold bi syndrome. BL-23 is the back shu point of the kidney, while GV-14 (Sea of qi) as the meeting point of the du meridian with the six yang channels acts to clear pathogenic factors from the exterior.

Meridian style treatment

Seem (1993) described the cutaneous regions of the body not simply as areas of musculoskeletal pain, but as surface projections of the underlying meridian pathways themselves. He claimed that in treating the cutaneous region the practitioner is in effect treating (albeit indirectly) underlying pathology. In this approach the body is divided into three zones, dorsal, lateral and ventral. The zones consist of the meridians running in the three circuits described on page 27, and shown in more detail in Table 4.4.

Table 4.4. Channels making up the cutaneous zones.

Zone	Yin	Yang	Yang	Yin	Extraordinary channels
Ventral	Lung	Large intestine	Stomach	Spleen	Conception vessel, penetrating vessel, yin linking vessel, yin motility vessel
Dorsal	Heart	Small intestine	Bladder	Kidney	Governing vessel and yang motility vessel
Lateral	Pericardium	Triple Energiser	Gallbladder	Liver	Girdle vessel and yang linking vessel

(Adapted from Seem, 1993)

The dorsal zone consists of the small intestine and bladder meridians (2nd circuit or tai yang) together with the governing vessel and the yang motility vessel. The area covered includes the forehead, top of the head, back, buttocks, posterior aspect of the legs and the outer edges of the feet (Fig. 4.4b). The corresponding yin vessels in the 2nd circuit are the heart and kidney.

The lateral zone encompasses the Triple Energiser and gallbladder channels (3rd circuit or shao yang) together with Girdle vessel (Dai mai) and the yin linking vessel (yin wei mai). This zone takes in the side of the head, the upper trapezius, upper back and latissimus dorsi, the side of the hip and the iliotibial band and the outer aspect of the lower leg and dorsum of the foot (Fig. 4.4c). The corresponding yin vessels in the 3rd circuit are the pericardium and liver.

The ventral zone consists of the large intestine and stomach channels (1st circuit or yang ming) together with the penetrating vessel (Chong mai), conception vessel (Ren mai), yin linking vessel (yin wei mai), and the yin motility vessel (yin qiao mai). Within this zone lie the face and neck, the dorsum of the arm to the index finger, the chest and anterior abdomen and the anterior aspect of the leg to the dorsum of the foot in the region of the second and third toes (Fig. 4.4a). The yin vessels of the 1st circuit are the lung and spleen.

The concept of treatment with meridian style acupuncture is firstly that in musculoskeletal treatment yang channels have a tendency towards excess and yin channels towards deficiency. In this case the channel is seen as yang and the Zang Fu organs as yin. There is therefore a deficiency in the constitution (core) of the individual and an excess in the symptoms (external). The approach parallels that of classical Japanese Acupuncture and emphasises the importance of the lungs, liver, spleen and kidneys as organs but pays little attention to the heart and pericardium.

The excess nature of the yang channels leads to cutaneous and myofascial constrictions in the involved zones, often identified as tender spots, trigger points or ahshi points. These trigger points are often linked in a specific order termed a Myofascial Chain (Seem, 1993) which mimics the meridian pathway (see also page 122). In treatment, both local and distal points are used to disperse the excess or *reduce the yang channels* and at the same time points are needled to support or *reinforce the yin channels* within the corresponding circuit. Going further, points on the upper body may be used to treat pain on the lower body and points on the left of the body to treat pain on the right. In the same way points on the back may be used to treat pain at the same level on the front of the body and internal points to treat external pains. In each case the opposite is also true, upper body points being used to treat lower body pain and lower body points for upper body pain, for example.

If we take chronic calf pain as a model, this pain exists in the dorsal zone. To treat this using meridian-style acupuncture we would reduce the dorsal zone yang vessels (locally the bladder and distally the small intestine) and reinforce the yin vessels, the kidney and possibly the heart (although in clinical practice the heart is rarely reinforced). Reduction and reinforcing may be achieved either by local needling techniques or by using sedation and tonification points. To bring in the appropriate extraordinary vessel associated with the dorsal zone

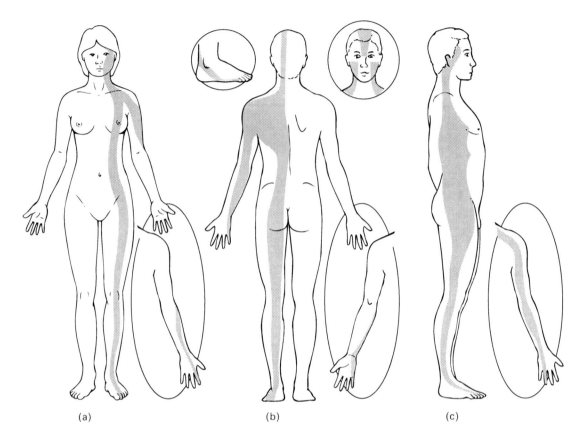

(a)   (b)   (c)

Figure 4.4. *Body zones used in meridian treatment.* (a) *Ventral zone;* (b) *dorsal zone;* (c) *lateral zone*

(Governing vessel and yang motility vessel) we can needle the confluence points SI-3 and BL-62.

Meridian sinews

The concept of meridian sinew treatment is an extension to that of meridian style acupuncture originally pioneered by Seem (1993). The meridian sinews lie superficially to the main meridians, but deep to the cutaneous regions, (see page 28), and follow the lines of the major muscles, tendons and ligaments (see Chapter 3). They all begin at the Jing Well points (Pirog, 1996) and travel proximally. They broadly follow the course of the main meridians but are wider (Deadman et al., 1998) (Fig. 4.5). They may be injured directly by external pathogens or trauma and are therefore of vital importance when treating musculoskeletal pain. The meridian sinews do not have specific points but their superficial nature makes them accessible to local needling of ahshi points. The main function of the meridian sinews is to carry defensive qi, and they do not connect to internal organs or have any internal effect. The meridian sinew can be seen to protect the main meridian from trauma and pathogenic attack (Pirog, 1996).

Meridian sinews have been described as responding to pathogenic attack on two levels (Pirog, 1996). During a level I disorder, the body has suffered an acute attack of trauma such as a recent sprain or strain, for example. Pathogenic qi enters the body and is immediately met by defensive qi coming out of the main meridian towards the surface of the body and the meridian sinew (Fig. 4.6a). This can be seen as an excess pattern where the meridian sinew is in excess and requires local shallow (5–20 mm) needling using a reducing technique to drain off the excess. As the defensive qi has come up from the main meridian, the main meridian is deficient and should be treated (possibly at a later treatment session) with a reinforcing technique and/or moxibustion, using distal points away from the injury site. The tonification (mother) point of the main meridian may be chosen as one suitable distal point. The symptoms here are of recent trauma, and superficial pain. Pain is made worse by minimal pressure and redness may be apparent on the body surface.

In the level II disorder the pathogenic attack has gone deeper and the external syndrome is moving internally (Fig. 4.6b). The defensive qi in the meridian sinew has been overcome and this leaves the sinew deficient. The pathogen is met with defensive qi in the main meridian now, but the response is weaker as the defensive qi is itself weakened. Treatment now aims at reinforcing the meridian sinew initially, using a reinforcing technique and/or moxa on the superficial painful points. The main meridian is reduced using a reducing technique and by needling the sedation (son) point. Because the condition is now moving internally, palpation may not be able to elicit specific pain and discomfort may now be more general. Where this is the case and a single meridian is difficult to distinguish as the source of pain, the luo-connecting point on the yin or yang aspect of the limb may be used.

Luo-connecting vessels

The luo-connecting vessels are superficial to the main meridian and form a network of fine vessels joining the yin and yang meridians and the internally/externally paired meridians. There use is especially important in cases of diffuse pain which involves both the inner and outer aspects of a limb and where two or more meridians are affected. Their structure is said to be tube-like (Pirog, 1996) and to include both blood vessels and lymphatic vessels. Their function is to collect pathogens, especially blood stasis and phlegm, which have overflowed from the main meridians. The luo vessels are visible (as opposed to the main meridians which remain invisible even when in excess) on the skin surface as tiny blood vessels filled with dark blood ('spider veins') or areas of local swelling. The luo vessels may be visualised as being blind ended with the closed end lying proximal. When the body is attacked by an external pathogen, the luo vessels fill and stagnation occurs causing palpable heat and pain (Fig. 4.7). The luo vessels are used to treat musculoskeletal conditions by draining them (traditionally bleeding the point) using a reducing technique.

The use of the luo vessels in cases where pain occurs over an area supplied by two paired channels gives the practitioner an additional

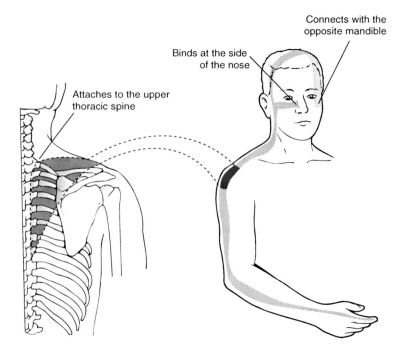

Figure 4.5. *Large intestine sinew channel. (Reproduced with permission from Deadman et al., 1998)*

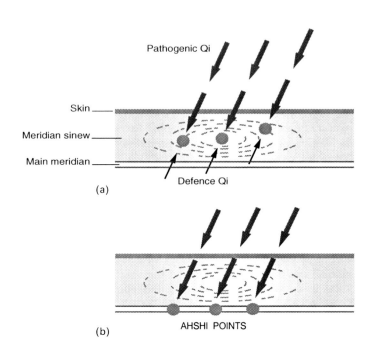

Figure 4.6. *Sinew channel reaction to pathogenic invasion. (a) Level I. External pathogen invades meridian sinew. Defensive qi moves out of main meridian to meet pathogen. Ahshi points superficial. (b) Level II. Pathogen moves inwards, and defence qi meets it in the main meridian. Ahshi points deeper. (Reproduced with permission from Pirog, 1996)*

method of treatment in particularly resistant cases. For example, in patients with lateral elbow pain, tender points are often found along the large intestine meridian, especially LI-11 together with periosteal points around the lateral epicondyle of the humerus. In cases where tender points are also found on the triple energiser and pericardium channels, the luo point of the most affected yang meridian channel is needled. In this example LI-6 would be chosen.

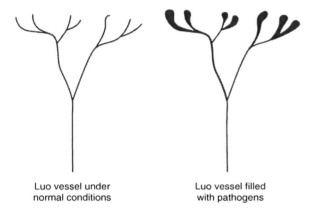

Luo vessel under
normal conditions

Luo vessel filled
with pathogens

Figure 4.7. *The luo vessels. (Reproduced with permission from Pirog, 1996)*

Acupuncture points

There are 361 standard acupuncture points or 'meridian points' which lie on the meridian channels themselves. The points on the 12 main meridians are symmetrical, while those of the GV and CV vessels lie on the midline only. In addition to the standard points there are 'extra' points which have specific locations and functions, but do not lie on meridians. Finally there are 'ahshi' points which do not have fixed locations but are determined by tenderness and pain.

Points have a variety of anatomical locations. Ten structures have been found in the close proximity to acupuncture points (Table 5.1). Nerves and changes in nerve direction and/or depth are particularly common as are structures such as tendons, joint capsules and fascial sheets which have a rich innervation. It has been claimed that some 80 per cent of acupuncture points correlate to perforations in the superficial fascia through which cutaneous nerves emerge (Heine, 1988). Others however argue that acupuncture points do not have exact locations (Mann, 1998) only 'areas of stimulation' which can be used to give therapeutic effects. In clinical practice the question obviously arises, how big are acupuncture points in diameter, and what is the margin of error when finding them? Many clinicians view acupuncture points as varying in size from 0.5–1.0 mm for nail points to 0.5–2.0 cm for points in large anatomical areas such as GB-30. There is also a general belief that acupuncture points represent a kind of 'vortex' with the point at its centre. To miss the point slightly is not to be totally unsuccessful, but to lessen the effect of needling.

The phenomenon of deqi may be used to home in on a point. Once the needle is inserted, if the patient fails to feel deqi, the needle may be partially withdrawn and its angle of insertion changed to maximise the deqi sensation. Acupuncture points have been shown to give significantly stronger needling sensation (deqi) when compared to sham points (Roth et al., 1997), so the use of deqi in point location may be useful.

It is interesting to note that although present day acupuncture charts in the west show precise anatomical positions of the points, traditional Chinese sources show only approximations to the point locations. There are probably a number of reasons for this. Firstly acupuncture in China was taught from Master to Pupil individually. To divulge too much detail would weaken the position of the Master. Secondly location of points would only have been taught practically rather than studied theoretically and so there would have been less need for charts. Finally, perhaps the more important theory is that point locations on charts are similar to those of trigger points. They are intended as a guide to where to start looking for the point (Seem, 1993). The practitioner must develop good palpatory skills to be able to locate areas of tissue tension change suitable for needling. This palpation skill is less stressed in western acupuncture, and this probably results in a poorer treatment outcome.

Table 5.1. Structures found close to acupuncture points.

Large peripheral nerves
Nerves emerging from a deep to a more superficial location
Cutaneous nerves rising from deep fascia
Nerves emerging from bone foramina
Motor points
Blood vessels in the vicinity of neuromuscular attachments
Along a nerve composed of fibres of varying size
Bifurcation point of a peripheral nerve
Richly innervated soft tissue (joint capsules, ligaments, fascial sheets)
Suture lines of the skull

(Dung, 1984)

Point categories

The acupuncture points situated on the meridian channels fall into a variety of categories.

The five shu points

The five shu points or 'transporting points' are situated at the ends of the limbs, at or below the elbow and knee (Table 5.2). Each of the points corresponds in TCM to the five phases or five elements (see chapter 1). The flow of the qi is said to begin or 'rise' at the well point (traditional name, 'jing-well'), build up in the spring (ying-spring) and stream (shu-stream) points and become 'abundant' at the river (jing-river) points. Finally, at the Sea (he-sea) point the qi is said to move deeper into the body and become 'flourishing' (Fig. 5.1).

The jing-well points are all (except KI-1) nail points, situated at the junction between lines drawn from the medial aspect of the nail and the nail base (Fig. 5.2). They are approximately 1 mm (0.1 cun) from the corner of the nail itself. The points were traditionally pricked to cause bleeding. Nowadays compression with a thin object such as the practitioner's finger nail or a pen top is normally used without breaking

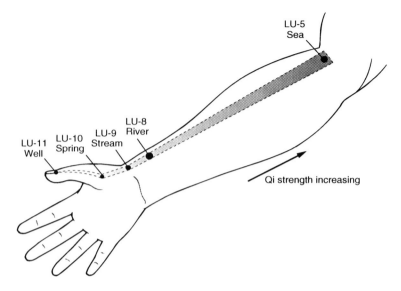

Figure 5.1. *The five shu (transporting) points of the lung channel*

the skin. The main function of jing-well points is to clear heat and restore consciousness. For example LU-11 may be used for an acute sore throat, and LI-1 for toothache. Most of the jing-well points may be used to bring a person around after fainting, but particularly LU-11. Because the jing-well points have no muscle covering, they are intensely painful to needle and are therefore not used frequently in modern acupuncture techniques. The jing-well point is located at the point where the yin and yang channels join, and the flow of qi begins. For this reason, they may be used for electrodiagnosis, measuring the activity of the channel at the nail point with a micro-volt meter.

Table 5.2. The five shu points and their correspondences.

Meridian	Jing-well Wood	Ying-spring Fire	Shu-stream Earth	Jing-river Metal	He-sea Water
YIN MERIDIANS					
Lung	11	10	9	8	5
Spleen	1	2	3	5	9
Heart	9	8	7	4	3
Kidney	1	2	3	7	10
Pericardium	9	8	7	5	3
Liver	1	2	3	4	8
YANG MERIDIANS	*Metal*	*Water*	*Wood*	*Fire*	*Earth*
Large intestine	1	2	3	5	11
Stomach	45	44	43	41	36
Small intestine	1	2	3	5	8
Bladder	67	66	65	60	40
Triple energiser	1	2	3	6	10
Gall bladder	44	43	41	38	34

The ying-spring points are said in TCM to clear heat from the upper portions of their respective meridian channels. For example SP-2 may

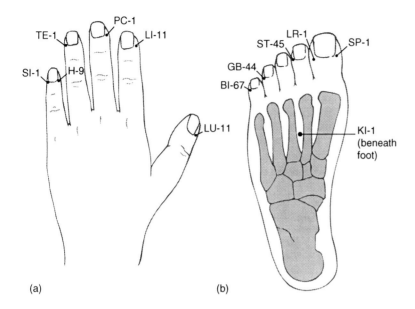

(a) (b)

Figure 5.2. *(a, b) Nail points of the hand and foot*

be used to clear heat and dampness from the spleen and stomach (its internally–externally connected channel) which has given rise to constipation and epigastric pain. KI-2 may be used to treat genital itching which results from failure of the kidney to clear heat. Heat is shown by fever and reddening of the body surface and the ying-spring points are traditionally used in cases where the face is flushed, the eyes red, and there is haemorrhage beneath the skin.

The shu-stream points correspond to the source points in the yin meridians (see below). The shu-stream points of the yang meridians are said to treat joint pain. Clinically they are normally only used for this function if they are local to a painful area, for example SI-3 and LI-3 when treating the finger joints.

The jing-river points are traditionally said to be used for cough and dyspnoea, but KI-7 is probably the most used in this respect. It is the tonification point of the kidney meridian and may be used to treat phlegm and oedema as one of the classic functions of the kidney organ in TCM is to 'regulate the water passages'. It works in conjunction with the spleen and lung organs to maintain water balance. From the point of view of musculoskeletal pain, an important feature of the jing-river points is their ability to treat diseases of the 'sinews and bones'. All the jing-river points are capable of doing this, but those of the yin meridians are most effective (Deadman et al., 1998). ST-41 may be used to treat painful obstruction syndrome due to damp in the leg, particularly the lower leg. SP-5 is an important point for heaviness and general pain in the joints. HT-4 is said to treat 'cold bones', and SI-5 to treat lockjaw. BL-60 is used extensively for spinal pain and is a heavenly star point. KI-7 in addition to its use with swelling, discussed above, may be used to treat the joints in general as the kidney organ dominates bone. GB-38 is used for 'invasion of wind' presenting as wandering joint pains. LR-4 may be used for contractions of sinews. Clinically BL-60, ST-41 and KI-7 are the most frequently used.

The He-Sea points are traditionally used to treat 'counter flow qi', that is qi which runs in the wrong direction in the meridian channel. Certainly the He-Sea points of the stomach and large intestines may have a harmonising effect, LI-11 and ST-36 being amongst the most widely used points in the body. Another more general use of the He-Sea points is to improve the passage of qi through a meridian. This becomes especially important in cases of painful obstruction syndrome. In these cases the He-Sea point may be used in addition to local points aimed at treating pain. For example, BL-40 may be used in the treatment of low back pain, and LI-11 in cases of frozen shoulder. Table 5.3 provides a synopsis of the clinical use of shu transport points.

Table 5.3a. Traditional usage of the shu transport points.

Jing-Well	'First aid' point
Ying-Spring	Clears heat in the body, and fever
Shu-Stream	Body heaviness and joint pain
Jing-River	Dyspnoea, cough and asthma
He-Sea	Qi flowing in wrong direction (counterflow)

Table 5.3b. Use of the shu transports points in treatment of Bi syndromes.

Jing-Well	Auxiliary point to release severe blockage or excess
Ying-Spring	Accelerates the flow of pathogens out of the meridian, often used with the shu stream point on yang meridians
	Treats heat, redness and swelling (heat bi syndrome)
	Treats severe painful (cold) bi syndromes where there is immobilisation of the joint
Shu-Stream	YANG MERIDIANS: bi syndromes in general, especially those characterised by exacerbation and remission
	YIN MERIDIANS: chronic (fixed) bi where primary pathogen is dampness, and bi patterns where there is core weakness especially for chronic knee or lower back pain
Jing-River	YANG MERIDIANS: bi syndrome with limb pain and spasm
	YIN MERIDIANS: primary treatment point for pain in yin meridians
He-Sea	Bi syndrome in yang meridians especially when pain is in the proximal region (shoulders, hip, neck, upper back) or if pain is associated with signs of bowel disease

(Adapted from Pirog, 1996)

Yuan source points

Each of the 12 meridians has a source point, said to be where the primary qi is housed (Table 5.4). These are located around the wrist or ankle. The source points are traditionally used to treat conditions affecting the relevant Zang Fu organ of the meridian channel. The source points are the 3rd point from the end of the channel in yin meridians. In the yang meridians they are the 4th point from the end, with the exception of the gallbladder channel where the source point is the 5th from the end. The yang source points are principally used to regulate the whole of the meridian channel, and to treat disorders along the channel length. For example, both LI-4 and SI-4 may be used to treat shoulder conditions depending on the area of pain. Clinically, the yang source points are found to have little effect on their corresponding Fu organs. The source points on the yin meridians however can be used to regulate the channel and can also have a noticeable effect on their corresponding Zang organ. For example LR-3 may be used to treat all conditions of the liver organ, and to treat pain (such as medial knee pain) along the liver channel.

Table 5.4. The Yuan source points.

Lung	LU-9	Bladder	BL-64
Large intestine	LI-4	Kidney	KI-3
Stomach	ST-42	Pericardium	PC-7
Spleen	SP-3	Triple Energiser	TE-4
Heart	HT-7	Gall bladder	GB-40
Small intestine	SI-4	Liver	LR-3

Luo-connecting points

The luo-connecting point (Table 5.5) is the point at which the exteriorly–interiorly linked meridians are joined, and is the starting point of the luo-connecting vessel. Luo-connecting points may therefore be used to move qi from a Zang organ to a Fu organ and vice versa. Clinically the point is often used to treat disorders involving both of the meridians and the area supplied by them. For example LU-7 may be used to treat neck pain even though the lung exterior channel only travels to the ribcage. Its internally–externally connected channel (the large intestine) does travel to the neck.

Table 5.5. The luo-connecting points.

Lung	LU-7	Bladder	BL-58
Large intestine	LI-6	Kidney	KI-4
Stomach	ST-40	Pericardium	PC-6
Spleen	SP-4	Triple Energiser	TE-5
Heart	HT-5	Gall bladder	GB-37
Small intestine	SI-7	Liver	LR-5

Xi-cleft points

Xi-cleft points (Table 5.6) are used to treat acute disorders of the corresponding organ or channel. Examples are the use of SI-6 as one of the points to treat acute shoulder pain when the patient is unable to tolerate local palpation or needling, and LU-6 to treat acute wheezing and asthma often combined with an extra point called Dingchuan lying 1 cun lateral to the depression below the spinous process of C7.

Table 5.6. The Xi-cleft points.

Lung	LU-6	Bladder	BL-63
Large intestine	LI-7	Kidney	KI-5
Stomach	ST-34	Pericardium	PC-4
Spleen	SP-8	Triple Energiser	TE-7
Heart	HT-6	Gall bladder	GB-36
Small intestine	SI-6	Liver	LR-6

Confluence points

The confluence points are eight points on the limbs where the primary meridians meet with the extraordinary meridians. They are used to bring the extra meridians into play (see page 2). Traditionally they are grouped into four groups of two points (see Table 3.5, page 45).

Influential points

There are eight influential points (Table 5.7), sometimes called the Hui-Meeting points. They are particularly useful when treating weak and elderly patients where the number of needles used has to be limited, and where there are multiple symptoms. A number of the points are used regularly. GB-34 the influential point for muscle and tendon is used when treating musculoskeletal disorders, and CV-17 the influential point for the respiratory system is often used in the treatment of asthma and chest conditions in general. LU-9 the influential point of the vascular system may be used with circulatory conditions such as intermittent claudication. CV-12 is normally only used for the stomach organ with a secondary effect on the large intestine. It is also the front mu point of the stomach and is used in most cases of epigastric pain, vomiting, and diarrhoea.

Table 5.7. The influential points.

Tissue and organ affected	Influential point
Zang organs	LR-13
Fu organs	CV-12
Respiratory system	CV-17
Blood	BL-17
Bone	BL-11
Bone marrow	GB-39
Muscle and tendon	GB-34
Vascular system	LU-9

Front mu and back shu points

There are 12 back shu and 12 front mu points (Table 5.8). The points may be used therapeutically, but also to aid diagnosis as they are said to become tender in response to conditions affecting their related Zang Fu organ. The back shu points are located along the inner bladder line. They correspond to the Zang Fu organs and other body regions that are more general such as the diaphragm and vital region shu. The back shu points are located at roughly the same level as their corresponding organ and western acupuncturists often describe them in terms of segmental effects. The front mu points are located on the chest or abdomen. Although both sets of points may be used to treat their related Zang Fu organ, clinically the back shu points are used more to treat conditions of the Zang organs and the front mu points to treat conditions of the Fu.

Table 5.8. Front mu and back shu points.

Zang Fu organ	Back shu point	Front mu point
Lung	BL-13	LU-1
Large intestine	BL-25	ST-25
Stomach	BL-21	CV-12
Spleen	BL-20	LR-13
Heart	BL-15	CV-14
Small intestine	BL-27	CV-4
Bladder	BL-28	CV-3
Kidney	BL-23	GB-25
Pericardium	BL-14	CV-17
Triple Energiser	BL-22	CV-5
Gallbladder	BL-19	GB-24
Liver	BL-18	LR-14

Tonification and sedation points

The tonification points ('mother' point) and sedation points ('son' point) increase and reduce the qi in a channel, respectively.

Each of the meridian channels corresponds to an element in the 5 element cycle (see page 12). For example the bladder meridian has *water* as its element. The element which comes before this in the five element cycle is *metal* and the element which comes after it is *wood*. The point which goes before an element is called the 'mother', the point which comes after it is called the 'son'. Each of the five shu points (see above) is attributed to one of the five elements as well. In the case of the bladder meridian the sequence is Metal (BL-67) water (BL-66) wood (BL-65) fire (BL-60) and earth (BL-40) (see Table 5.2, page 64). The element point of the bladder channel (water) is then BL-66 while the mother point (metal) is BL-67 and the son point (wood) is BL-65. These two points would therefore be used to tonify and sedate activity in the meridian.

Sedation points may be needled in cases of excess conditions affecting a meridian. Tonification points are used in cases of deficiency of a meridian, often in association with moxibustion or warm needling. For example, chest conditions with coughing are normally related to the lung organ, and so points along this meridian may be needled. If a patient shows a cough, frequent colds and a weak 'croaky' voice it would suggest *deficiency* of the lungs. The tonification point of the lung channel (LU-9) may therefore be needled. On the other hand, a patient with a heavy cough who is producing copious phlegm and presents with a 'full' feeling in the chest is likely to have an *excess* condition of the lungs. In this case the sedation point of the lung channel (LU-5) can be used. The tonification and sedation points are listed in Table 5.9.

Table 5.9. Tonification (mother) and sedation (son) points.

Meridian	Tonification point	Sedation point
Lung	9	5
Large intestine	11	2
Stomach	41	45
Spleen	2	5
Heart	9	7
Small intestine	3	8
Bladder	67	65
Kidney	7	1
Pericardium	9	7
Triple Energiser	3	10
Gallbladder	43	38
Liver	8	2

Heavenly star points and command points

The heavenly star points and the command points are two groups of points which are used extensively in the treatment of musculoskeletal conditions. The heavenly star points (Table 5.10) were first described by an important Chinese physician named Ma Dan-yang. The command points (Table 5.11) were originally a group of four points which was extended to a group of six. Again these points are attributed to a single individual, this time named Gao Wu. These points should always be considered as additional points to supplement (and increase the effectiveness) of musculoskeletal acupuncture treatments.

Table 5.10. The heavenly star points and their use in musculoskeletal conditions.

LU-7	Headache, especially when one-sided
LI-4	Headache and facial pain
LI-11	Elbow pain
ST-36	Stomach pain, knee pain
ST-44	Chills in the hands and feet
HT-5	Heaviness of the body
BL-40	Lumbar pain radiating to the knee
BL-57	Lumbar pain radiating to the calf
BL-60	Lumbar pain radiating to the foot
GB-39	Painful obstruction syndrome (fixed bi)
GB-34	Painful obstruction syndrome (cold bi)
LR-3	Symptoms associated with stress and anxiety

Table 5.11. The command points and their use in musculoskeletal treatment.

ST-36	Abdomen
BL-40	Lumbar region
LU-7	Head and nape of neck
LI-4	Face and mouth
PC-6	Chest and lateral costal area
GV-26	Resuscitation (digital pressure only)

Description of commonly used acupuncture points

Lung channel

Lu-7

On the radial aspect of the forearm approximately 1.5 cun proximal to the centre of the anatomical snuffbox (Figs 5.3 and 5.4). In the cleft between the tendons of brachioradialis and abductor pollicis longus. To locate the point, place the forefinger in the snuffbox and run it

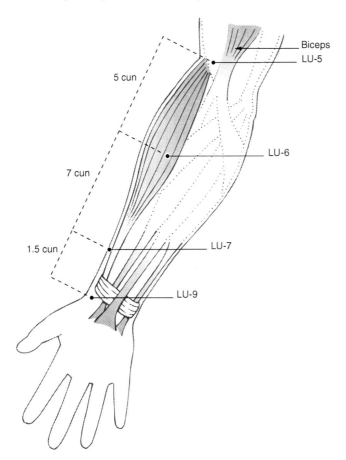

5 cun

Biceps
LU-5

7 cun

LU-6

1.5 cun

LU-7

LU-9

Figure 5.3. *Lung points on the forearm*

proximally along the shaft of the radius. The finger will fall into the cleft between the two tendons. Traditionally you can 'shake hands' with your patient, interlocking the thumb and forefinger web space. Your forefinger lies on top of the patient's radius, and will fall naturally into the approximate position of LU-7.

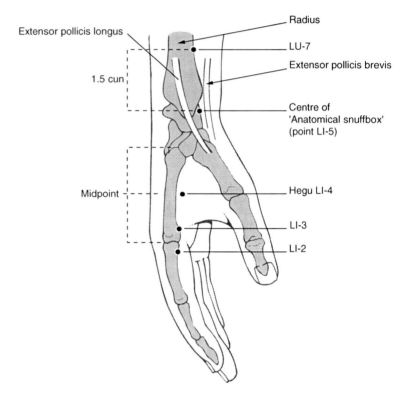

Figure 5.4. *Large intestine points on the hand*

Needling: Pinch up a single skin fold and needle transversely 0.5–1.0 cun. The cephalic vein and the superficial ramus of the radial nerve lie close to this point.

LU-5

At the cubital crease of the elbow, to the radial side of the biceps tendon (Fig. 5.3). Flex the elbow to 90° and needle with the elbow flexed to avoid the cubital vein. The point lies lateral to the tendon rather than right next to it.

Needling: Perpendicular insertion 0.5–1.0 cun depending on the patient's build.

LU-9

At the transverse crease of the wrist joint in the depression to the medial (ulnar) side of the tendon of abductor pollicis longus (Figs 5.3 and 5.18). This point lies lateral to the radial artery. LU-9 is at the same level as HT-7 which lies at the lower border of the pisiform bone.

Needling: Perpendicular, 0.3–0.5 cun.

LU-6

Lies on a straight line from LU-5 at the elbow to LU-9 at the radial wrist crease, 5 cun distal to LU-5 (Fig. 5.3). If the distance between LU-5 and LU-9 is divided into half, LU-6 lies 1 cun *proximal* to the midpoint.

Needling: Perpendicular to a maximum depth of 1.5 cun.

Large intestine

LI-4

Between the 1st and 2nd metacarpal bones on the dorsum of the hand (Fig. 5.4). Located at the midpoint of the 2nd metacarpal close to the radial border. When the patient adducts the thumb to the forefinger, the point lies at the level with the end of the skin crease close to the 1st metacarpal bone. Traditionally the transverse crease of the distal interphalangeal joint of the right thumb is lined up with the web between the thumb and forefinger of the left. The point then lies at the tip of the right thumb.

Needling: Perpendicular insertion 0.5–1.0 cun.

LI-10

Lies on a line connecting LI-11 (radial side of the elbow crease) and LI-5 (centre of the anatomical snuffbox). LI-10 is 2 cun distal to LI-11, (Fig. 5.5).

> **Clinical note**
>
> Cases of tennis elbow can occur at four major sites. The first is to the common extensor origin over the lateral epicondlye of the humerus at the attachment of extensor carpi radialis brevis. The second is to the supracondylar ridge of the humerus at the attachment of extensor carpi radialis longus. Thirdly the musculo-tendinous junction between the tendon and extensor muscles may be affected, and finally the extensor muscle belly's themselves may be the source of pain. LI-11 lies medial to the common extensor origin and is more likely to be effective as a local point in cases where the extensor origin or supracondylar ridge is affected. Where the muscle belly itself is affected, choose LI-10.

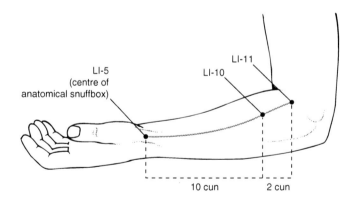

Figure 5.5. *Large intestine points on the radial aspect of the forearm*

Needling: Perpendicular insertion to a maximum depth of 1.5 cun.

LI-11

At the radial side of the elbow crease, midway between the tendon of biceps and the lateral epicondyle (Fig. 5.5). Locate the point with the elbow flexed.

Needling: Perpendicular insertion 1.0–1.5 cun.

LI-14

The point lies slightly superior to the insertion of the deltoid muscle (the deltoid tuberosity of the humerus) on a straight line joining LI-15 and LI-11 when the arm is abducted to 90° (Fig 5.6).
Needling: Oblique insertion 1.0–1.5 cun.

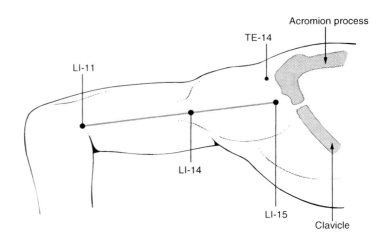

Figure 5.6. *Large intestine points on the lateral aspect of the shoulder*

Clinical note

When the arm is abducted, action of the deltoid tends to pull the head of the humerus up into the sub-acromial arch increasing the risk of tissue impingement. To counteract this pull, the subscapularis and infraspinatus contract to pull the humerus in towards the glenoid fossa and downwards away from the sub-acromial arch. This is due to the angle of pull of these muscles whose fibres run supra-laterally. As abduction proceeds, the head of the humerus is pulled beneath the acromion at 90° abduction creating a fossa. At the anterior aspect of this fossa lies LI-15, at the posterior aspect TE-14. Needling these points is therefore helpful in cases of impingement pain of either the long head of biceps or the supraspinatus.

LI-15

In the depression anterior and inferior to the acromion when the arm is abducted to 90° (Fig 5.6.). Slightly anterior to the bundle of the medial fibres of the deltoid muscle.
Needling: Perpendicular insertion directed to the centre of the axilla to a depth of 1.0–1.5 cun if the arm is abducted. Where the patient is unable to abduct the arm insertion may be transverse oblique directed distally.

LI-16

On the superior aspect of the shoulder, in the depression between the acromion process and the lateral 1/3rd of the clavicle (Fig. 5.21)
Needling: Oblique insertion posteriorly 0.5–1.0 cun. In thin patients there is a risk of pneumothorax if a deep perpendicular insertion is used.

LI-18

On a line level with the laryngeal prominence (Adam's apple) between the sternal and clavicular heads of the sternomastoid muscle, approximately 3 cun from the prominence (Fig. 5.7).
Needling: Oblique insertion 0.5 cun.

Stomach

ST-6

In the centre of the belly of the masseter muscle, approximately 1 cun anterior and superior to the angle of the jaw (Fig. 5.8).
Needling: Perpendicular 0.5 cun.

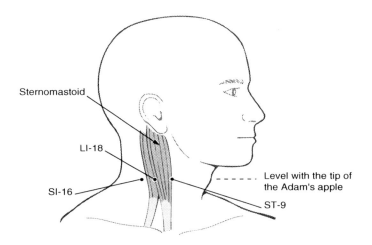

Figure 5.7. *Points on the neck level with the Adam's apple*

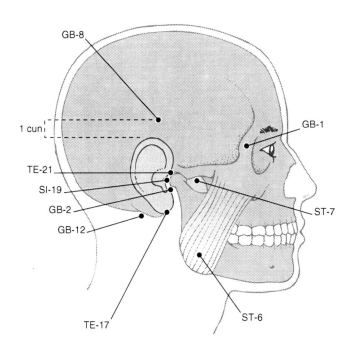

Figure 5.8. *Points on the side of the head*

ST-7

In the depression anterior to the condyloid process of the mandible (Fig. 5.8). Ask the patient to open their mouth and the condyloid process will move forward and outwards making it easier to palpate. As the mouth is closed again keep the finger on the same skin position and the condyloid process will slide back to its original position. The finger now rests in the depression over ST-7.

Needling: Perpendicular 0.5 cun.

Clinical note

There are five abdominal points in line with the umbilicus. CV-8 lies in the centre of the umbilicus. The next four points lie on the horizontal line of the umbilicus, at a distance from the midline. From the midline KI-16 is positioned 0.5 cun laterally, ST-25 2.0 cun laterally. SP-15 is on the umbilicus line at the lateral edge of rectus abdominis and GB-26 at the point of intersection between the horizontal umbilical line and a vertical line drawn down from the free end of the 11th rib (Fig. 5.9).

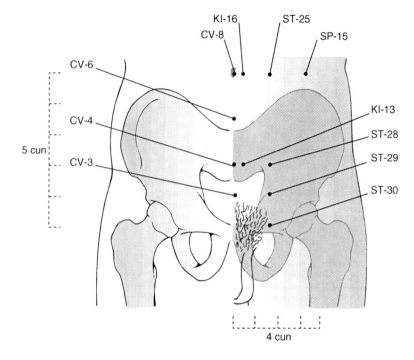

Figure 5.9. *Points on the lower abdomen*

ST-25

On the abdomen 2 cun lateral to the umbilicus (CV-8) in the middle of the rectus abdominis muscle belly (Fig. 5.9).
Needling: Oblique insertion 1.0 cun.

ST-31

On the upper leg at the junction of a line drawn down from the anterior superior iliac spine and a line draw across from the lower border of the symphasis pubis (Fig. 5.10). The horizontal level may also be taken through the apex of the greater trochanter.
Needling: Perpendicular 1.0–2.0 cun.

ST-32

On a line joining the lateral border of the patella and the anterior superior iliac spine, 6 cun proximal to the superior border of the patella (Fig. 5.10). If the distance between the superior border of the patella and the apex of the greater trochanter is devided into thirds, this point lies approximately at the junction of the upper 2/3rd and lower 1/3rd.
Needling: Oblique insertion 1.0–2.0 cun.

ST-34

On a line joining the lateral border of the patella and the anterior superior iliac spine, 2 cun proximal to the superior border of the patella (Fig. 5.10).
Needling: Oblique insertion 1.0–1.5 cun.

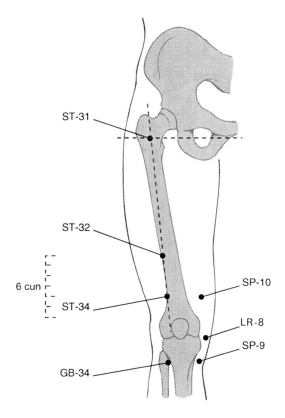

Figure 5.10. *Points on the anterior thigh*

ST-35

This point is the lateral of the two Xiyan points, the 'eyes of the knee'. It lies in the hollow lateral to the patella tendon when the knee is flexed (Fig. 5.11).

Needling: Perpendicular insertion to a depth of 1.0–2.0 cun directed towards the centre of the knee.

ST-36

3 cun (1 hand-breadth) inferior to ST-35 and one finger-breadth lateral to the anterior crest of the tibia (Fig. 5.11). This point lies below and medial to GB-34. Place the palm of the hand over the patient's patella and the tip of the middle finger with fall onto the tibial crest. The point lies one finger-breadth lateral to this point.

Needling: Perpendicular 1.0–1.5 cun.

ST-38

On the shin, midway between the popliteal crease and the lateral malleolus, one finger-breadth from the anterior crest of the tibia (Fig. 5.12).

Needling: Perpendicular 1.0–1.5 cun

Clinical note

Stomach points are commonly used to treat knee and thigh pain. ST-35 and ST-34 may be used as local points for knee joint pain, while ST-34 and ST-32 may be used as local points for pain in the rectus femoris muscle. ST-31 is a commonly used local point for hip pain especially hip arthritis. The three points ST-31, ST-36, and ST-41 may be used to treat disorders affecting the whole leg such as hemiplegia.

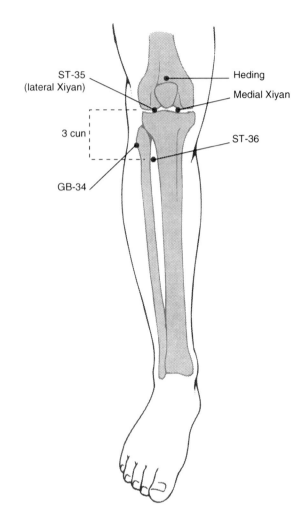

Figure 5.11. *Points in relation to the patella*

ST-40

On the shin, midway between the popliteal crease and the lateral malleolus, two finger-breadths from the anterior crest of the tibia (Fig. 5.12).
Needling: Perpendicular 1.0–1.5 cun.

ST-41

On the dorsum of the ankle approximately in the middle of a line drawn from the apex of the lateral malleolus (Fig. 5.13). The point lies between the tendons of extensor hallucis longus and extensor digitorum longus. If the patient extends the big toe against resistance, the tendon of extensor hallucis will stand out. ST-41 can then be located lateral to the tendon.
Needling: Perpendicular insertion to 0.5 cun.

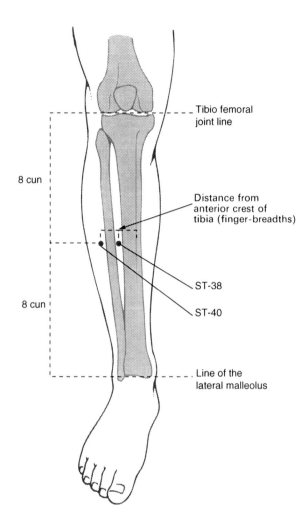

Tibio femoral joint line

8 cun

Distance from anterior crest of tibia (finger-breadths)

ST-38

8 cun

ST-40

Line of the lateral malleolus

Figure 5.12. *Stomach points near the central tibia*

ST-44

On the dorsum of the foot, between the 2nd and 3rd toes. The point lies 0.5 cun proximal to the web space (Fig. 5.13).

Needling: Perpendicular or oblique angled proximally 0.5 cun.

Spleen

SP-4

On the medial aspect of the foot, distal and inferior to the base of the 1st metatarsal bone (Fig. 5.14). The point lies in a depression formed by the edge of the tendon of tibialis anterior.

Needling: Perpendicular or oblique 0.5–1.0 cun.

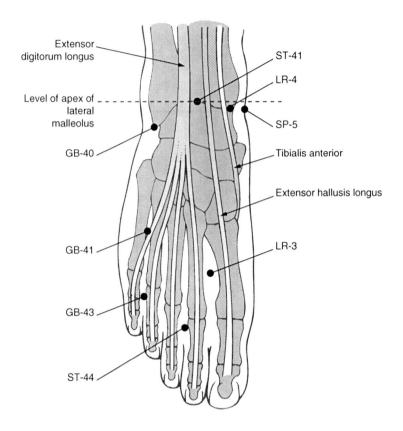

Figure 5.13. *Points on the dorsum of the foot*

SP-5

On the medial aspect of the foot at the junction of lines drawn along the anterior border and inferior border of the medial malleolus (Fig. 5.14).
Needling: Perpendicular or oblique 0.3 cun.

SP-6

On the medial aspect of the shin 3 cun (one hand-breadth) superior to the apex of the medial malleolus (Fig. 5.14). The point lies in a shallow depression towards the posterior aspect of the tibia. This point is contraindicated in pregnancy as it is said to induce labour.
Needling: Perpendicular 1.0–1.5 cun.

SP-9

On the medial aspect of the knee, in the depression between the medial condyle of the tibia and the posterior border of the tibia, (Figs 5.15 and 5.10). Palpate by running the finger up the posterio-medial border of the tibia until it reaches the condyle.
Needling: Perpendicular 1.0–1.5 cun.

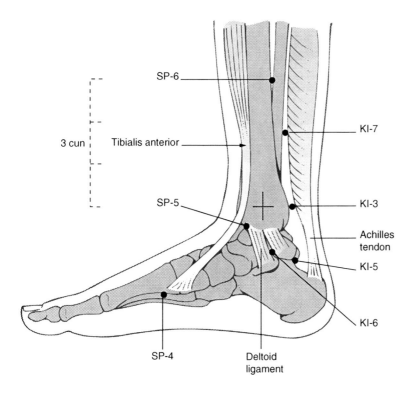

Figure 5.14. *Points on the medial aspect of the foot*

SP-10

2 cun above the superior border of the patella, in the centre of the vastus medialis obliqus (VMO). The height of the patella is 2 cun, so this point is one patella length above the superior border of the patella itself (Fig. 5.10).

Needling: Perpendicular or oblique insertion 1.0–1.5 cun.

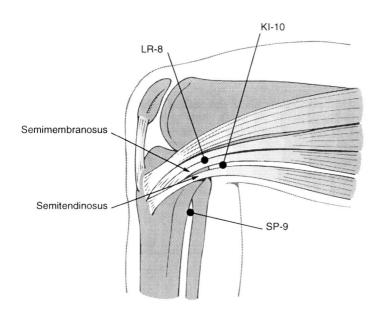

Figure 5.15. *Points on the medial aspect of the knee*

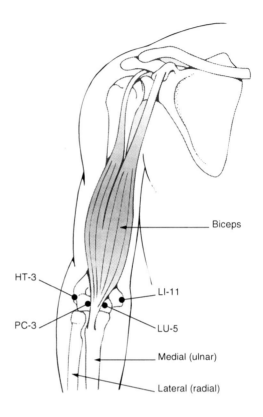

Figure 5.16. *Points on the cubital crease*

Heart

HT-3

At the medial end of the elbow crease when the joint is fully flexed. Midway between the tendon of biceps and the medial epicondyle (Fig. 5.16).

Needling: Oblique insertion 0.5–1.0 cun.

HT-7

On the transverse crease of the palmar aspect of the wrist (Fig. 5.17). Locate the point at the wrist joint in the depression at the proximal border of the pisiform bone. The point lies to the radial side of flexor carpi ulnaris. To aid location, palpate the ulna and slide your finger along its shaft towards the wrist until the finger comes into contact with the pisiform bone.

Needling: Oblique insertion 0.5–0.8 cun.

Small intestine

SI-3

On the ulnar aspect of the hand at the head of the 5th metacarpal bone

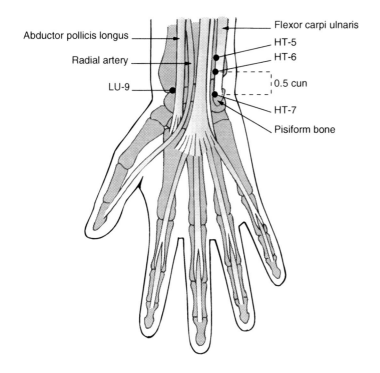

Figure 5.17. *Points on the palmar aspect of the wrist*

(Fig. 5.18). When a loose fist is made the point may be located at the junction of the red and white skin. The point should be needled with the fingers relaxed.

Needling: Perpendicular or oblique 0.5 cun.

SI-6

On the dorsum of the wrist, in a shallow depression to the radial aspect of the high point of the ulna styloid (Fig. 5.19). Palpate by placing the finger on the highest point of the ulna styloid and sliding the finger radially. Pronate and supinate the forearm to bring the depression into prominence.

Needling: Oblique insertion 0.5 cun.

SI-8

Between the tip of the olecranon process of the ulna and the medial epicondyle of the humerus (Fig 5.20).

Needling: Oblique insertion 0.3–0.5 cun.

SI-9

1 cun superior to the posterior axillary crease when the arm is held by the side (Fig. 5.21).

Needling: Perpendicular 1.0–1.5 cun.

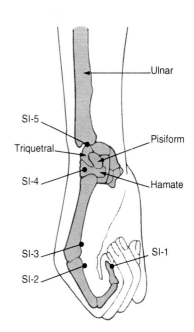

Figure 5.18. *Points on the ulnar aspect of the wrist and hand*

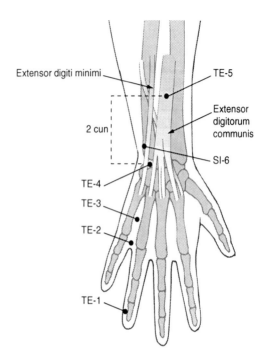

Figure 5.19.*Triple Energiser points on the dorsum of the wrist and hand*

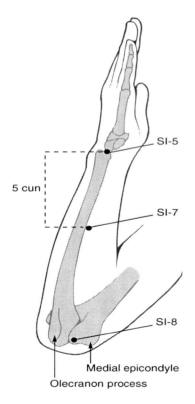

Figure 5.20. *Principle small intestine points of the forearm*

SI-10

On the posterior aspect of the shoulder directly above SI-9 in line with the posterior axillary crease, when the arm hangs by the side (Fig. 5.21). The point is palpated in the depression inferior to the scapular spine (acromion angle) over the head of the humerus. Slide the finger up vertically from the axillary crease until it rests in the depression.

Needling: Perpendicular 1.0–1.5 cun.

SI-11

This point forms the apex of an equilateral triangle with SI-9 and SI-10. If a line is drawn from the inferior angle of the scapula to the mid-point of the scapular spine, SI-11 lies at the junction between the upper 1/3rd and the lower 2/3rd of this line (Fig. 5.21).

Needling: Perpendicular 0.5–1.5 cun.

SI-12

Directly above SI-11 in the centre of the suprascapular fossa. This point lies in the centre of a depression when the arm is raised to 90° abduction (Fig. 5.21).

Needling: Oblique insertion 0.5–1.0 cun.

SI-19

On the side of the head directly in front of the tragus of the ear (Fig. 5.21). When the mouth is open and the condyloid process slides forwards, this point lies in the centre of the depression which is formed. TE-21 is directly above this point, GB-2 directly below.

Needling: Perpendicular 0.5 cun.

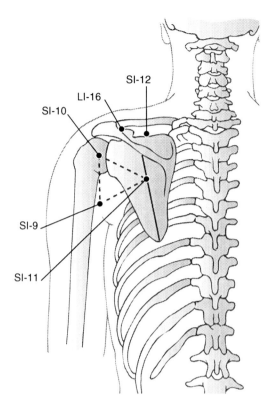

Figure 5.21. *Small intestine points on the posterior aspect of the shoulder*

Bladder

BL-2

At the medial end of the eyebrow directly above the inner canthus of the eye (Fig. 5.22). This point lies in the centre of a depression at the medial end of the supraorbital ridge.

Needling: Transverse insertion directed towards the centre of the

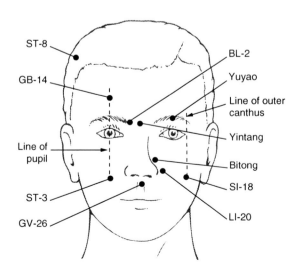

Figure 5.22. *Major points on the face*

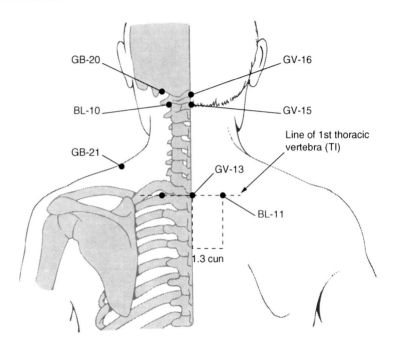

Figure 5.23. *Points on the lower neck*

eyebrow (yuyao extra point) for supraorbital pain or to the inner canthus (BL-1) for eye disorders.

BL-10

1.3 cun lateral to the 1st cervical vertebra (C1). To locate this point first find the external occipital protuberance (point GV-16) and C1 lies 0.5 cun down from this point (GV-15). BL-10 is lateral to this point by nearly 1.5 cun, lying over the transverse process of C1 (Fig. 5.23).
   Needling: Perpendicular 0.5–0.8 cun.

BL-11

1.5 cun lateral to the 1st thoracic vertebra (T1). To locate T1, lie the patient in prone, propped up on their elbows (elbow support prone lying) and first locate C7 and T1 as the most prominent central bumps at the base of the neck. Ask the patient to rotate the neck and C7 will move from side to side, T1 will remain fixed (Fig. 5.24).
   Needling: Oblique insertion towards the spine 0.5–1.0 cun.

BL-23 to BL-26

These points lie 1.5 cun lateral to the midline at the level of the lower border of the spinous processes of the 2nd to 5th lumbar vertebra (L2–L5). The points lie at the apex of the erector spinae muscle and should be needled if painful to palpation (Fig. 5.24).
   Needling: Oblique insertion towards the spine 1.0–1.5 cun.

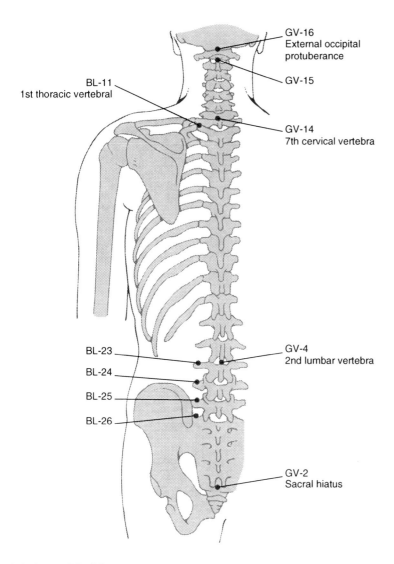

GV-16
External occipital
protuberance

GV-15

BL-11
1st thoracic vertebral

GV-14
7th cervical vertebra

GV-4
2nd lumbar vertebra

BL-23

BL-24

BL-25

BL-26

GV-2
Sacral hiatus

Figure 5.24. *Points of the back*

BL-27 to BL-30

The points lie approximately 1.5–2.0 cun lateral to the midline at the level of the 1st to 4th sacral foramen (Fig. 5.25). Note that the sacral foramen are in a line drawn from the lumbo-sacral (LS) junction to the sacro-coccygeal hiatus. If the hand is placed on this line each of the four finger-tips of one hand should lie on one foramen. The second sacral foramen (BL-28) lies at the mid-point of the line joining the LS junction and the hiatus.

Needling: Perpendicular insertion 0.5–1.0 cun.

BL-32

Over the second sacral foramen (Fig. 5.25). Approximately at the midpoint of a line joining the posterior superior iliac spine (PSIS) and the sacro-coccygeal hiatus.

Needling: Perpendicular (with a slight medial oblique angle) through the foramen 1.0–1.5 cun.

> **Clinical note**
>
> All acupuncture points may be used clinically if they are painful to palpation. In the case of the points on the inner bladder line, in addition to local pain many are also back shu points relating to general body functions or organs. If painful to palpation they are often diagnostic (from a TCM perspective) and again should be needled. As the bladder points are positioned at the apex of the erector spinae muscle, this line should be massaged using deep finger kneading to establish if pain relates to specific points.

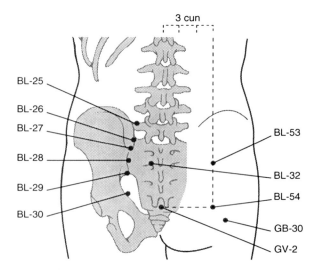

Figure 5.25. *Points on the lower lumbar spine and sacrum*

Clinical note

BL-36/37 and 40 all lie between the hamstring muscles. These points are traditionally used in cases of low back pain referred into the leg. In addition however they can also be of use to reduce pain and spasm in the hamstring muscles after tearing, and can be used to relax the muscles prior to stretching. In this later case they are needled with the patient lying on his/her side to enable straight leg stretching (when the needles are removed) without changing the body position. In addition BL-39 may be needled in cases of tendonitis of the biceps femoris.

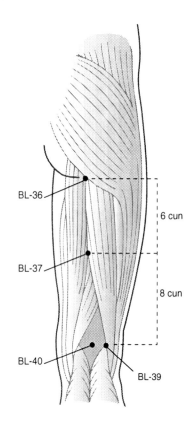

Figure 5.26. *Points on the posterior thigh*

BL-36

In the centre of the transverse gluteal crease directly above the centre of the popliteal fossa (BL-40)(Fig. 5.26).
Needling: Perpendicular 1.0–2.0 cun.

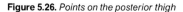

BL-37

In the centre of the thigh 6 cun below BL-36 (Fig 5.26).
Needling: Perpendicular 1.0–2.0 cun.

BL-39

At the lateral edge of the popliteal crease, just medial to the tendon of biceps femoris (Fig. 5.26).
Needling: Perpendicular 1.0 cun.

BL-40

In the centre of the popliteal crease, in the depression midway between the tendons of biceps femoris and semitendinosus. This point is best located with the knee slightly flexed (Fig. 5.26).
Needling: Perpendicular or oblique 1.0 cun (the popliteal artery lies directly below this point).

BL-54

In the buttock, 3 cun (1 hand-breadth) lateral to the sacro-coccygeal hiatus (Fig. 5.25).
Needling: Perpendicular 1.5–2.5 cun.

BL-57

Between the bellies of the gastrocnemius muscle at the midpoint of a line joining the popliteal fossa (BL-40) and the lateral malleolus (BL-60) (Fig. 5.27).
Needling: Perpendicular 1.0–1.5 cun.

BL-60

On the lateral aspect of the ankle, in the centre of the depression between the apex of the lateral malleolus and the achilles tendon (Fig. 5.27).
Needling: Perpendicular 0.5–1.0 cun.

BL-62

On the lateral aspect of the ankle, 0.5 cun inferior to the apex of the lateral malleolus. This point lies in the depression below the peroneal tendons (Fig. 5.28).
Needling: Oblique insertion 0.3–0.5 cun.

Kidney

KI-3

In the depression between the apex of the medial malleolus and the achilles tendon (Fig. 5.14). This point lies level with the malleolar apex and is opposite to BL-60.
Needling: Perpendicular 0.5–1.0 cun.

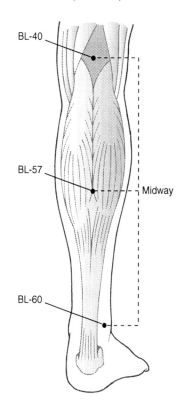

Figure 5.27. *Major bladder points of the calf*

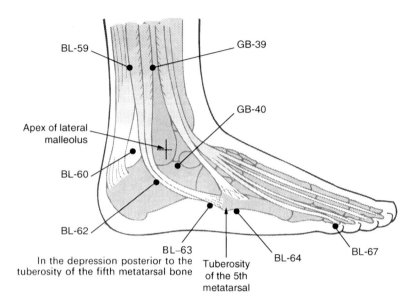

Figure 5.28. *Points on the lateral aspect of the ankle*

KI-5

Anterior and superior to the calcaneal tuberosity (Fig. 5.14). This point lies in the depression at the site of the insertion of the Achilles tendon into the calcaneum, 1 cun below KI-3.

Needling: Oblique or perpendicular insertion away from the bone 0.3–0.5 cun.

KI-6

1 cun below the prominence of the medial malleolus (Fig. 5.14). This point lies in the groove between the two major bundles of the deltoid ligament (the anterior and posterior tibiotalar bands).

Needling: Oblique insertion 0.3–0.5 cun directly towards the malleolus.

KI-7

On the anterior border of the achilles tendon on a line 2 cun above the apex of the medial malleolus (KI-3) (Fig. 5.14).

Needling: Perpendicular 0.5–1.0 cun.

KI-10

At the medial end of the popliteal crease between the tendons of semitendinosus and semimembranosus (Fig. 5.15). This point lies about 1 cun posterior and slightly inferior to LR-8.

Needling: Perpendicular 1.0–1.5 cun.

Clinical note

Kidney points are used extensively for treatment of the Achilles tendon. KI-3 and KI-5 may be used for injury to the teno-osseous junction of the tendon while KI-7 may be used for the musculo-tendinous junction. KI-6 may be used to treat injury to the deltoid (medial) ligament of the ankle. This injury may occur traumatically but is more usually seen in cases of hyperpronation and 'flat feet'. In this latter case a taping must be used to hold the calcaneum in its neutral position and take the stretch off the ligament between treatment sessions.

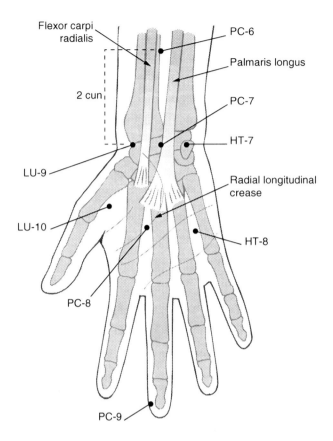

Figure 5.29. *Points on the palm of the hand*

Pericardium

PC-3

On the ulnar side of the transverse cubital crease to the side of the biceps tendon (Fig. 5.16). The point is best located with the elbow slightly bent. Have the patient perform lightly resisted elbow flexion and supination to cause the biceps tendon to stand out.

Needling: Perpendicular 0.5–1.0 cun.

PC-6

On the flexor aspect of the forearm, 2 cun proximal to the wrist crease (PC-7) (Fig. 5.29). The point lies between the tendons of palmaris longus and flexor carpi radialis. Directly over the median nerve.

Needling: Perpendicular or oblique insertion 0.5–1.0 cun.

PC-7

At the wrist crease between the tendons of palmaris longus (sometimes absent) and flexor carpi radialis (Fig. 5.29). Directly over the medial nerve. The point is level with HT-7 (base of the pisiform) and LU-9.

Needling: Oblique insertion 0.3–0.8 cun.

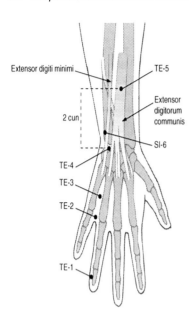

PC-8

When a loose fist is formed this point lies at the tip of the 3rd finger at the point on contact with the radial longitudinal crease of the palm (Fig. 5.29). The point lies between the 2nd and 3rd metacarpal bones at the radial side of the 3rd.

Needling: Perpendicular 0.5 cun (or use of acupressure).

Triple Energiser

TE-2

0.5 cun back from the margin of the web between the 4th and 5th fingers (Fig. 5.20). Locate and needle with the hand formed into a loose fist.

Needling: Perpendicular 0.5 cun.

TE-3

On the dorsum of the hand between the 4th and 5th fingers (Fig. 5.20). The point lies just proximal to the metacarpophalangeal joint.

Needling: Perpendicular 0.5 cun.

TE-4

On the dorsum of the wrist level with the wrist crease (Fig. 5.20). In the depression between the tendons of extensor digitorum communis and extensor digiti minimi (extend the wrist and fingers to make these tendons stand out, and then relax the hand before needling). Locate the point by sliding the palpating finger in a line between the 4th and 5th finger until it rests in the depression.

Needling: Oblique insertion 0.5 cun.

TE-5

2 cun proximal to the wrist crease (TE-4) between the radius and ulna (Fig. 5.20). The point lies to the radial side of extensor digitorum communis and this tendon may have to be pressed to the side to facilitate needling.

Needling: Oblique insertion 0.5 cun.

TE-10

1 cun proximal to the apex of the olecranon when the elbow is flexed (Fig. 5.30).

Needling: Perpendicular 0.5–1.0 cun.

TE-14

Posterior to the acromion. When the arm is abducted to 90° this point is in the posterior depression next to the acromion (Fig. 5.6 and Fig. 5.30). LI-15 lies in the anterior depression.

Needling: With the arm abducted, perpendicular insertion 1.0–1.5 cun. With the arm held by the side, transverse-oblique insertion (towards the elbow) 1.5 cun.

Figure 5.30. *Points on the posterior aspect of the upper arm*

TE-17

Behind the earlobe (fold the lobe forwards to needle) in the depression between the ramus of the mandible and the mastoid process (Fig. 5.31).
Needling: Perpendicular 0.5–1.0 cun.

TE-21

In the depression anterior to the supratragic notch (Fig. 5.8). This point lies slightly superior to the condyloid process of the mandible (SI-9).
Needling: Needle with the mouth open (close when needle is in place) oblique insertion slightly posterior 0.5 cun.

Gallbladder

GB-2

In the hollow below the intertragic notch (Fig. 5.8). This point lies in a vertical line with TE-21 at the top, SI-19 in the middle and GB-2 at the base. The point is more easily located with the mouth open to accentuate the hollow.
Needling: Slightly posterior insertion 0.5–1.0 cun.

GB-8

1 cun directly above the apex of the ear (Fig. 5.31). The point lies in a slight depression.
Needling: Transverse insertion 0.5 cun directed towards the area of pain. Insert through the skin and into the subcutaneous areolar tissue next to the skull. More shallow insertion into the skin only is painful.

GB-12

In the shallow depression posterior and inferior to the mastoid process (Figs 5.8 and 5.31). Palpate by placing the finger directly over the apex of the mastoid process, then slide backwards along the ridge of bone until the finger rests in the depression.
Needling: Oblique insertion directed inferiorly 0.5 cun.

GB-14

1 cun above the centre of the eyebrow (yuyao, *extra point* lies in the centre of the eyebrow) directly above the pupil (Fig. 5.22).
Needling: Pinch up the skin and needle transversely 0.5 cun.

GB-20

Below the occiput (close to the skull) approximately midway between the external occipital protruberance (GV-16) and the mastoid process (Fig. 5.23). This point lies in the hollow between the attachment of sternomastoid and the trapezius.
Needling: Oblique insertion directed either inferiorly or towards the nose 0.5–1.0 cun.

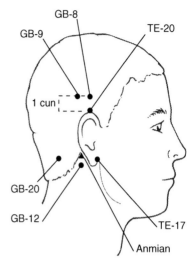

Figure 5.31. *Points in relation to the ear*

Clinical note

Three major structures attach to the ASIS; the sartorius muscle, the external oblique, and the inguinal ligament. The sartorius may suffer from injury to the teno-periosteal junction or complete avulsion of its insertion onto the ASIS. The external oblique, most noticeably the lateral (vertical) fibres may also tear at the teno-osseous junction on the ASIS. Groin disruption, which involves a separation (dehiscence) of the conjoint tendon from the inguinal ligament may also occur in footballers especially (Norris, 1998). Each of these conditions may benefit from needling GB-27 or GB-28 if these points are painful. In addition periosteal needling of the ASIS itself may also give some relief (see page 154). When some pain relief has been obtained, light exercise therapy may be begun with the aim of stretching and remodelling the developing scar tissue.

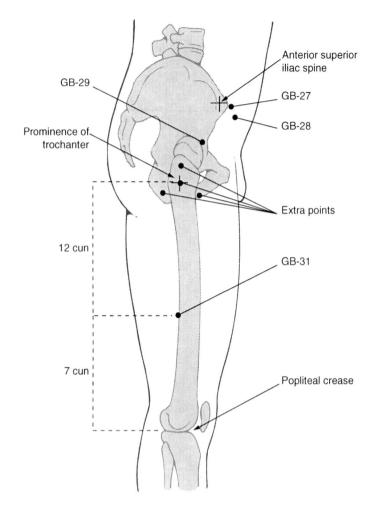

Figure 5.32. *Points on the lateral aspect of the hip*

GB-21

Midway between the spinous process of the 7th cervical verebrae (GV-14) and the tip of the acromion process (Fig. 5.23). This point is normally tender to palpation and is located at the highest part of the crest (in a sagittal plane) of the muscle.

Needling: Squeeze up the muscle and use an oblique insertion 0.5–1.0 cun directed posteriorly.

GB-27/28/29

There are several points around the hip joint which are of use in hip arthritis in particular (Fig. 5.32). GB-27 lies in the depression just anterior (medial) to the anterior superior iliac spine (ASIS). GB-28 lies slightly medial to GB-27. GB-29 is at the midpoint of a line drawn between the ASIS and the apex of the greater trachanter. A number of extra points may be found in relation to the greater troachanter (see page 99)

Needling: GB-27/28 may be needled perpendicularly 0.5–1.0 cun, GB-29 perpendicularly 1.0–2.0 cun.

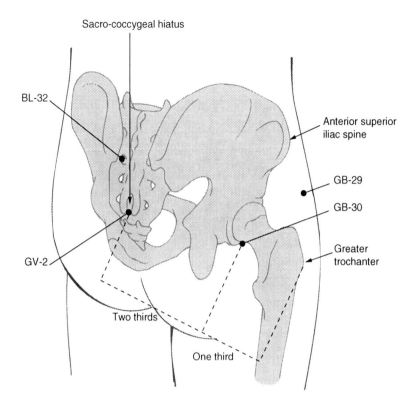

Sacro-coccygeal hiatus

BL-32

Anterior superior
iliac spine

GB-29

GB-30

GV-2

Greater
trochanter

Two thirds

One third

Figure 5.33. *Points over the buttock*

GB-30

One third of the distance between the sacro-coccygeal hiatus (GV-2)
and the apex of the greater trochanter (Fig. 5.33).

Needling: Perpendicular insertion 2.0 cun. The point is best located
and needled with the patient lying on their side with the knee and hip
flexed (1/2 crook side lying), knee resting on a pillow.

GB-31

On the lateral aspect of the thigh within the ilio-tibial band (Figs 5.32
and 5.34). This point lies 12 cun inferior to the apex of the greater
trochanter. The distance between the greater trachanter and the knee
crease is 19 cun. If this distance is divided in thirds (just over 6 cun
each) the point lies 1 cun proximal to the junction of the upper 2/3rd
and the lower 1/3rd. The point may be found by asking the patient to
reach down their side while standing. The tip of the middle finger
roughly approximates to this point in this position.

Needling: Perpendicular insertion 1.0–2.0 cun.

GB-33

On the lateral side of the knee in the depression between the upper edge
of the lateral epicondyle of the femur and the biceps femoris muscle
(Fig. 5.34).

Needling: Perpendicular 1.0 cun.

Clinical note

Friction syndromes of the ilio-tibial band (ITB) are common in endurance sports. They can occur at the upper end of the ITB over the greater trochanter or at the lower end over the epicondyle. GB-33 may be used as a local point for ITB friction syndrome around the knee and extra points over the greater trochanter for ITB friction syndrome over the hip. GB-31 may be used where pain and tightness occur in the ITB itself (see page 158).

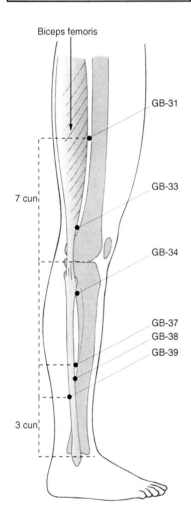

Figure 5.34. *Major gallbladder points of the leg*

GB-34

1 cun anterior and 1 cun inferior to the apex of the head of the fibula (Fig. 5.34). To locate the head of the fibular slide the fingers up the shaft of the fibula from the shin. The apex is the most prominent point (not the most anterior point).

Needling: Perpendicular 1.0–1.5 cun.

GB-37

On the lateral aspect of the lower leg 5 cun superior to the apex of the lateral malleolus (Fig. 5.34). The point lies approximately at the junction of the upper 2/3rd and lower 1/3rd of a line joining the lateral malleolus and the popliteal crease.

Needling: Perpendicular 1.0 cun.

GB-39

3 cun superior to the apex of the lateral malleolus, between the posterior border of the fibula and the peronei (Fig. 5.34).

Needling: Perpendicular 1.0 cun. Press the peronei away from the fibula and insert the needle into the groove which is formed. A slightly posterior insertion is used to avoid striking the periosteum of the fibula.

GB-40

In the depression anterior and inferior to the lateral malleolus (Fig. 5.28). The point is located at the junction of lines drawn anterior and inferior from the borders of the malleolus.

Needling: Perpendicular or oblique insertion 0.5–1.0 cun.

GB-41

In the depression distal to the space between the 4th and 5th metatarsal bones (Fig. 5.13). The point lies lateral to the tendon of extensor digitorum longus (EDL). If the finger is run up between the 4th and 5th toes it will pass over the EDL tendon to rest in a shallow depression, in which the point lies.

Needling: Perpendicular 0.5–1.0 cun.

Liver

LR-3

On the dorsum of the foot in the hollow distal to the junction of the 4th and 5th metatarsals (Fig. 5.13). To locate the point run the finger up the web between the 4th and 5th toes until it rests in the hollow.

Needling: Perpendicular 0.5–1.0 cun angled slightly towards the centre of the foot.

LR-8

Superior to the medial end of the popliteal crease, between the tendons of semimembranosus and semitendinosus (Fig. 5.16). Locate the point by flexing the knee to identify the end of the popliteal crease. Then, flex the knee against resistance to make the hamstring tendons stand out. The semitendinosus is the more prominent of the two tendons.

Needling: Perpendicular 1.0–1.5 cun.

Conception vessel

CV-3

On the midline, 1 cun superior to the symphasis pubis (CV-2), 4 cun inferior to the umbilicus (CV-8) (Fig. 5.9).

Needling: Oblique insertion 0.5 cun.

CV-6

On the midline, 2 cun superior to the symphasis pubis (CV-2), 3 cun inferior to the umbilicus (CV-8) (Fig. 5.9).

Needling: Oblique insertion 0.5 cun.

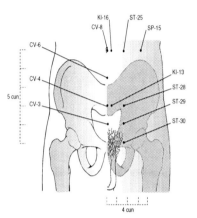

CV-8

In the centre of the umbilicus (Fig. 5.9). Do not needle this point, use moxibustion only.

CV-12

On the midline, 4 cun above the umbilicus (Fig. 5.35). The point is between the umbilicus (CV-8) and the sternocostal angle (CV-16).

Needling: Perpendicular or oblique insertion 0.3–0.8 cun.

CV-16

On the midline, at the sternocostal angle (Fig. 5.35).

Needling: Transverse insertion 0.5 cun directed inferiorly along the midline.

CV-17

On the midline at the level of the 4th intercostal space, approximately between the nipples in the male (Fig. 5.35).

Needling: Transverse insertion 0.5 cun.

CV-22

On the midline in the centre of the suprasternal fossa (jugular notch) (Fig. 5.35).

Needling: Transverse/oblique insertion 0.3 cun (into the skin only) or perpendicular insertion 0.2 cun, then direct the needle along the inner surface of the sternum. *This latter method of needling must not be attempted without special training and close clinical supervision.*

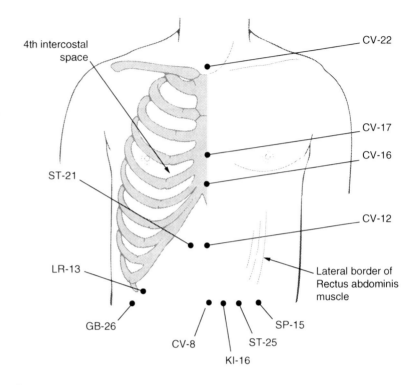

Figure 5.35. *Conception vessel points of the chest*

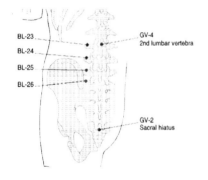

Governor vessel

GV-2

On the midline, in the sacro-coccygeal hiatus (Figs 5.24 and 5.33).
Needling: Oblique insertion 0.5 cun directing the needle superiorly.

GV-4

On the midline below the spinous process of the 2nd lumbar vertebra (L2) (Fig. 5.24). Note that a line joining the crest of the two ilia corresponds approximately to the body of L4, and is therefore level with the lower border of the L3 spinous process.
Needling: Perpendicular or oblique insertion 0.5 cun. Note that the spinal canal lies approximately 1.5 cun deep to the skin surface, but this measurement will vary with stature.

GV-14

On the midline in the depression below the spinous process of the 7th cervical vertebra (C7) (Fig. 5.24).
Needling: Perpendicular or oblique insertion 0.5 cun.

GV-16

On the midline in the depression below the external occipital protuberance (Figs 5.23 and 5.24).
Needling: Perpendicular or oblique insertion 0.5–1.0 cun directed inferiorly.

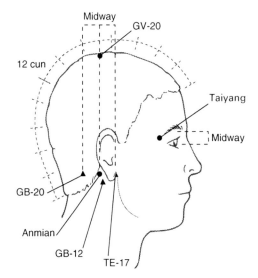

Figure 5.36. *Extra points on the side of the head*

GV-20

At the vertex of the head, approximately at the meeting point of a line joining the apex of each ear (Fig. 5.36). The distance between the anterior and posterior hairlines is 12 cun, on a sagittal line. GV-20 is measured as 5 cun away from the anterior hairline and 7 cun away from the posterior hairline.

Needling: Transverse insertion 0.5 cun.

GV-26

Above the upper lip, at the junction of the upper 1/3rd and lower 2/3rd of the philtrum (Fig. 5.22).

Needling: Oblique insertion 0.3 cun or use strong finger pressure for resuscitation.

Extra points

Greater Trochanter

There are several points around the greater trochanter (Fig. 5.32) which may be used successfully in painful hip conditions especially arthritis. A single point may be found over or slightly below the apex of the trachanter (Low, 1987), which may be needled perpendicularly 0.5 cun. In addition, three points may be used surrounding the trachanter, one superior and the other two anterior and posterior (Ellis et al., 1994). These may be needled to a depth of 1.5–2.0 cun perpendicular or slightly oblique pointing inwards. Moxibustion is of particular value.

Xiyan

Below the patella in the hollows on either side of the patella tendon when the knee is flexed (Fig. 5.11). These points lie directly over the patella fat pads. The lateral Xiyan point is ST-35.

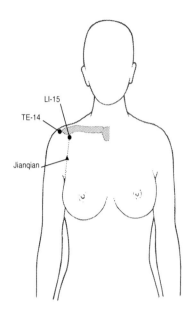

Figure 5.37. *The extra point Jianqian*

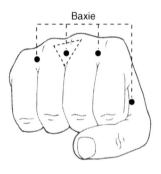

Figure 5.38. *Baxie extra points*

Needling: Perpendicular 1.0–1.5 cun directed towards the centre of the knee joint. Needle these points with the knee flexed and supported over a rolled pillow.

Heding

At the midpoint of the superior border of the patella (Fig. 5.11).
Needling: Perpendicular or oblique 0.5 cun.

Jianqian

On the anterior aspect of the shoulder midway between the anterior crease of the axilla and LI-15 (Fig. 5.37).
Needling: Perpendicular 1.0–1.5 cun or oblique insertion downwards 1.5–2.0 cun.

Anmian

Behind the ear, midway between GB-20 and SJ-17, slightly superior and posterior to GB-12 (Fig. 5.31).
Needling: Perpendicular 0.5 cun.

Yintang

Directly between the eyebrows (Fig. 5.22).
Needling: Pinch up a skin fold and use a transverse insertion 0.5 cun directed inferiorly.

Yuyao

In the centre of the eyebrow directly above the pupil when the subject is looking forward (Fig. 5.22).
Needling: Transverse 0.5 cun.

Baxie

When a fist is made the points lie in the depressions between the metacarpal heads (Fig. 5.38). Each point lies proximal to the web margins. The points lie in the centre of a triangle formed by the metacarpal heads and the web margin.
Needling: Perpendicular insertion 0.5 cun directed along the line of the metacarpal shafts.

Taiyang

Over the temple in the depression 1 cun posterior to the midpoint of a line joining the lateral end of the eyebrow with the outer canthus of the eye (Fig. 5.36).

6

Patient questioning and point selection

Patient questioning

Subjective examination or 'patient questioning' (inquiring) is a very important part of the initial acupuncture treatment session. It steers the practitioner towards the selection of specific meridians and ultimately specific points. The aim is to determine firstly the *nature of the disorder* in terms of the eight principles especially, and secondly the likely *Zang Fu organ* affected.

Questions are formatted into six categories as in Table 6.1. The answers to the questions may not be cut and dry, but together with other forms of examination they contribute to the total picture of the disorder. As we question the patient we must try to discover whether the condition is yin/yang, hot/cold, deficient/excess, or internal/external. In addition, recognising the function of the Zang Fu organs we are trying to ascertain which organ is likely to be giving rise to the symptoms. Determination of the organ involved is often dependent both on individual symptoms, and on organising a number of these symptoms into meaningful groups.

Hot and cold symptoms give information about the depth of the disease particularly. The presence of chills (shivering) and fever (high temperature) together suggests that the body surface has been invaded by a pathogen and the body is countering the invasion with anti-pathogenic qi. The body is therefore fighting, and winning. If the patient has a fever, but not chills, it suggests that the pathogen is beginning to win the fight and moving from the exterior to the interior of the body. The patient has an aversion to heat, and may throw the bedclothes off. They sweat profusely and have a marked thirst. This is similar to a cold changing to flu, for example. Where shivering (chills) occur without fever, the syndrome is interior cold of the deficiency type. In other words there is a deficiency of yang and the body needs to be warmed with moxibustion, for example. For musculoskeletal treatment the importance of hot/cold aversion and preference lies mainly in the bi syndrome (see page 54). Patients with chronic conditions often show an aversion to cold and symptom exacerbation in cold weather. This indicates that they would benefit from heat, in some form, as part of the management of their condition. This could take the form of warm needling, infra-red therapy or simply using a hot water bottle and wrapping up warm in cold weather, for example.

Table 6.1. Questions for patients receiving acupuncture.

Cold and Hot *Recently have you:*
1. Had a fever (temperature)?   Yes/No
2. Had chills (shivering)?   Yes/No
3. Felt cold and wanted to keep warm?   Yes/No
4. Had chills and a fever together?   Yes/No

Sweating *Recently:*
5. Do you sweat more profusely than normal?   Yes/No
6. Do you feel sweaty most of the time?   Yes/No
7. Do you suddenly break out in sweat?   Yes/No
8. Are you very sweaty at night?   Yes/No

Appetite, Thirst And Taste *Recently:*
9. Is your appetite better or worse than normal?   *Please circle as appropriate*
10. Are you more often thirsty than you were?   Yes/No
11. Do you crave certain foods?   Yes/No
12. Do you particularly dislike certain foods?   Yes/No
13. Do you have a bitter/sour taste in your mouth?   *Please circle as appropriate*
14. Is your mouth more often dry than it was?   Yes/No
15. Is your mouth more often very sticky?   Yes/No

Stools And Urine
16. Are you constipated?   Yes/No
17. Are your stools loose/watery/bloodstreaked?   *Please circle as appropriate*
18. Is your urine clear/light yellow/dark yellow/light red?   *Please circle as appropriate*
19. Do you dribble urine occasionally?   Yes/No

Pain
19. Does your pain move from one part of the body to another?   Yes/No
20. Is your pain of sharp or pricking nature?   Yes/No
21. Do you have pain with a heavy feeling in the body?   Yes/No
22. Do you have pain with muscle spasm?   Yes/No
23. Is your pain burning/cold/dull (in nature)? *Please circle as appropriate*

Sleep *Recently:*
24. Do you sleep well through the whole night?   Yes/No
25. Do you have poor sleep and dizziness during the night?   Yes/No
26. Is your sleep disturbed, do you wake up several times?   Yes/No
27. Do you have difficulty falling asleep, but eventually sleep through?   Yes/No

Sweating (perspiration) tells us about the body's ability to control its protective surface. The yang of daytime should change to yin at night. When this does not occur, there is a deficiency of yin and a proportional hyperactivity of yang. This presents as night sweats. Spontaneous sweating (insensible sweating in western terms) shows that qi is no longer controlling the opening and closing of the sweat pores, and qi is deficient. Profuse sweating coinciding with fever, thirst and a desire for cold drinks shows heat internally almost as if the cold drinks are needed to 'put out the fire' in the body.

Appetite, taste and thirst give information about the spleen and stomach in particular in terms of digestion. A poor appetite in a prolonged illness shows weakness of the stomach and spleen. Where there is a feeling of abdominal bloating qi stagnation is present in these organs. If the appetite is excessive, the food is being 'burnt' by excess stomach fire. In the same vein thirst indicates either consumption of body fluids ('burning') or use of body fluids in swelling or phlegm. Alteration in taste may be relevant taken alongside other symptoms. A bitter taste implicates the gallbladder, a sweet taste with a sticky mouth the spleen and stomach and a sour taste the liver and stomach. In clinical practice the bitter bile taste of the gallbladder is more reliable than the others.

Defecation and urination give information about the bladder and bowels as well as the stomach and spleen. Constipation with dry stools shows an accumulation of heat while loose stools shows a cold condition with the spleen being the affected organ. When the urine is excessively yellow heat is said to be present. An increased volume of urine implicates both the kidney and bladder organs while painful urination (as with cystitis) suggests 'damp heat' in the bladder. Dribbling of urine again suggests the kidney and bladder organs, this time through qi deficiency.

Pain is possibly the most important factor when questioning the patient with a musculoskeletal problem. The *site* and *nature* of the pain both being important. The site of pain indicates the meridian (or meridian sinew) affected and the nature of pain helps to identify the pathogen. Moving pains suggest *wind*, heavy pains *damp*, and burning pains *heat*. For more details on pain see Chapter 4.

Patterns of sleep are important for the heart and liver especially. In TCM the mind/spirit is split into five aspects. The mind (shen) is housed by the heart. The ethereal soul (hun) by the liver and the corporeal soul (po) by the lungs (see also page 16). The ethereal soul could be translated as 'spirit' in western terms while the corporeal soul is that part of the spirit which remains in the body after death. The intellect (yi) is housed by the spleen and the will-power (Zhi) by the kidneys. In mental/emotional problems all of these organs may have an affect. For more details of TCM in mental health see Maciocia (1994) pp. 197–280. Insomnia with dizziness implicates the heart and spleen while generally restless sleep suggests the heart organ and fire.

For female patients, questions about menses and leukorrhea (mucous secretion from the vagina) are also important. A shortened cycle with excessive flow which is thick and deep red in colour indicates heat while a lengthened cycle with a profuse flow indicates cold. Thin and scanty flow indicates blood deficiency while an irregular cycle suggests disharmony. With leukorrhea, deficiency and cold is seen with a watery profuse flow, excess and heat with a reduced thick flow. The spleen, liver, and kidney meridians are usually indicated with menstrual disorders.

Traditional methods of diagnosis

Pulse diagnosis

There are several forms of pulse diagnosis in TCM. In this book the most basic form is presented to allow the practitioner to have at least an

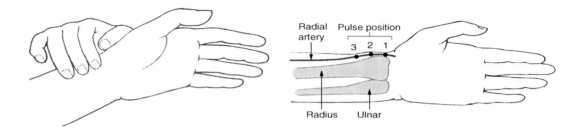

Figure 6.1. *Pulse examination in TCM. (Reproduced with permission from Kaptchuk, 1983)*

appreciation of this technique. To gain competence with pulse diagnosis prolonged practice under close supervision is required. Because pulse diagnosis is so skilled, electrodiagnosis is becoming more popular with western acupuncturists. The two combined can contribute much to meridian selection in particular.

Pulse diagnosis in its basic form can give information about meridian differentiation and the nature of a disease. To take the pulse the patient is positioned sitting in front of a table. Their hand is placed on a small cushion or folded towel with the wrist in slight extension and ulnar deviation. The therapist's middle finger is placed next to the inner aspect of the patient's radial styloid. The pulse is felt at three levels called cun (distal), guan (middle) and chi (proximal). On the left hand these relate to the heart, liver and kidney, respectively, on the right hand to the lung, spleen and kidney (Fig. 6.1). The guan area is opposite the radial styloid and felt with the middle finger, the cun with the forefinger and the chi with the ring finger. The fingers are gently rounded so that the pads feel the pulse. The fingers should be placed slightly apart for a tall patient and further together if the patient is short.

Ensure that the same horizontal level is maintained for each finger and the pressure used is the same for each. Press on each point, first lightly and then more heavily, to differentiate the *depth*, *speed*, *strength* and *shape* of the pulse.

The depth of the pulse is either superficial or deep. A superficial pulse is easy to feel, (with minimal finger pressure), a deep pulse can only be felt by pressing hard. A superficial (thin or floating) pulse is seen in external conditions, a deep pulse in interior conditions. The speed of the pulse is fast or slow. A slow pulse, defined as being less than four beats per breath indicates cold syndromes, a fast pulse, defined as more than five beats per breath indicates heat. The strength of the pulse indicates deficiency and excess. A weak (empty) pulse shows deficiency, and strong (full) pulse excess.

Several pulse shapes are seen but are difficult to differentiate without in-depth training. Descriptions such as thready, rolling, hesitant, string-taut, and knotted are used to indicate more clearly the nature of a condition.

Tongue diagnosis

Tongue diagnosis is another method of differentiating syndromes in TCM. On the whole it is less subjective than pulse diagnosis. Many of the meridians or their branches have connections directly to the tongue. A branch from the heart meridian travels to the root of the tongue (the heart 'opens to the tongue'), while the spleen meridian travels to the root and spreads over the lower surface of the tongue. The kidney meridian terminates at the root of the tongue. The various organs are attributed to specific regions of the tongue (Fig. 6.2). The tip reflects changes to the heart/lungs, the sides the liver/gallbladder, the centre the spleen/stomach, and the root the kidneys. For descriptive purposes the tongue is divided into the tip, central portion, root (back) and border.

When the tongue is observed we look at the general shape of the tongue itself (the tongue body) and the coating which covers the tongue sometimes called the 'moss'. The tongue coating is produced by stomach qi and reflects the condition of the stomach. A normal tongue should be slightly red with a thin white coating. It should be slightly moist but not dry or greasy.

When looking at the tongue body, a pale coloration indicates deficiency or cold syndromes and a red tongue body shows excess or heat. A blue/purple tongue or blue spots indicates blood stagnation (stasis). When the tongue body is swollen and therefore larger than normal it shows damp and fluid retention. Where tooth marks are present because the tongue appears too big for the mouth, the spleen (or sometimes the kidney) is affected. A thin tongue indicates deficiency. Cracking on the tongue indicates heat-consuming body fluids and shows yin deficiency.

Changes in the coating of the tongue reflect dysfunction of the yang organs, especially the stomach. A thin coating exists where the tongue body can be seen through the coating. The coating is thick if the tongue body cannot be seen through the coating at all. A thin coating indicates that a pathogenic factor is attacking the exterior portion of the body. As the condition becomes more serious and internal the coating becomes thicker. Retention of damp, phlegm or food shows as a thick coating. The moisture content of the coating shows the condition of the body fluid. A normal coating is moist. If the coating is dry it indicates that the body fluid is being consumed. If there is no coating the tongue is said to be 'peeled' and this shows the stomach is affected and its qi and yin have been consumed. Excessive moisture and dribbling indicates upward movement of damp and cold.

The colour of the coating also gives information. A yellow tinge shows heat, and white, cold. Where the coating is grey or black the condition is chronic and has been present for a prolonged period.

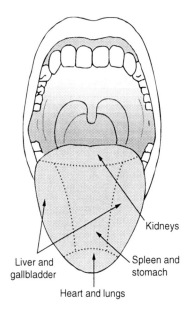

Kidneys

Liver and gallbladder

Spleen and stomach

Heart and lungs

Figure 6.2. *Regions of the tongue*

Acupuncture channel differentiation

Questioning the patient, and tongue/pulse diagnosis if it is used, helps to indicate the Zang Fu organ that is likely to be affected. The position of pain helps to indicate the meridian affected. Also from the examination we gain information about the nature of the disease from the point of view of the eight principles. In musculoskeletal conditions we are really only concerned to know if the condition is external or internal, hot or cold, excess or deficient. If a condition is external, local points on the meridian may be used to alleviate pain. Internal conditions may involve points in addition to treating the organ affected. Where a condition is cold, heat such as moxibustion or warm needling is used. Where a hot condition is present, points to 'drain' the excess heat are used. An excess condition requires needling of the sedation (son) point and/or a reducing method of needling. A deficient condition requires reinforcing needling (see Chapter 7) and/or needling of the tonification (mother) point of the meridian.

Identification of pathogens other than heat and cold is important in bi syndromes especially (see Chapter 5). Where wind is present points (such as LI-11, GB-21) may be used to release this. Similarly where damp is present this must be addressed with points such as SP-9, for example.

Some of the most commonly used Acupuncture points

There are 361 acupuncture points in current usage, and in addition to these there are an infinite number of ahshi points. Not all are relevant to the practice of musculoskeletal therapy but some are more important and more generally used than others. The aim of this section is to highlight the points more commonly used in everyday practice. That is not to say that others are not important, indeed they are, but they will be met less often.

Although this book deals with musculoskeletal conditions, general conditions seen alongside these in an outpatient department or private practice are also mentioned. Musculoskeletal symptoms (especially when chronic) rarely occur in isolation, and mentally linking these conditions with others that the patient is suffering from will often give a better guide to appropriate treatment. Much of the information for this section comes from Pirog (1996) and Deadman et al. (1998) to which the reader is referred for further information.

Lung

The lung is the most superficial of the yin meridians and as such it is vulnerable to invasion by external pathogens. The meridian begins internally in the middle jiao in the region of the stomach. It is this reason that makes the lung meridian important in treating firstly vomiting due to rebellious stomach qi, and secondly diarrhoea and abdominal distension. In these cases LU-5 (he-sea point) is used to assist the descending function of both the lung and stomach. LU-6 (xi-cleft point) may be effectively used to treat blood in the sputum or 'splitting blood' (haemoptysis) and is often combined with BL-17, the influential point for blood for this purpose.

The lung goes only to the throat and its energy is deeper than that of its internally/externally paired meridian the large intestine. For this reason the lung tends to be used to treat symptoms of the lower respiratory tract (coughing) while the large intestine is used to treat those of the upper respiratory tract (sinus congestion).

Because the lung organ is the upper source of water in the body (the lung regulates the water passages), the lung meridian is important in the treatment of urinary disorders. In these cases LU-7 is often used. LU-9 (source point) is the major point for relieving cough, and it is said to 'transform phlegm'. Using this point with self-administered acupressure may also be effective. As the source point and tonification point of the lung meridian, LU-9 is very useful in cases of chronic cough, wheezing and shortness of breath due to deficiency and may be combined with the extra point Dingchuan ('Calm Dyspnoea') which lies up to 1.0 cun lateral to the depression below C7. In addition it is often combined with CV-17, the influential point of the respiratory system.

Large intestine

The large intestine is a yang meridian which is typically in excess and often suffers from heat. The meridian is associated with disorders of the upper respiratory tract (especially sinuses), eyes and head. In fact the large intestine meridian is the most important of the yang meridians with reference to pain in the head and face, with typical conditions affecting the sinuses, gums, eyes, and teeth. It is important in the treatment of shoulder pain with LI-15 being an important local point for this purpose.

Of all the large intestine points, LI-4 (source point) must surely be the most important. It is said that this point tends to open the meridians of the upper body and push the qi up and out. Both LI-4 and LI-11 are essential points to disperse wind (wind heat or wind cold), and are especially useful in painful shoulder conditions. Attack by an external pathogen will affect the lung as it is the most exterior organ. The large intestine can be viewed as an exterior reflection of the lung (its coupled meridian). Because the lungs control the skin and hair, attack by an external pathogen will affect the external portion of the lung. This type of condition can therefore be treated by needling large intestine points (Deadman et al., 1998). When clearing wind, LI-4 may therefore also be combined with LU-7, although the affect is mostly on the upper body. Wind clearance for the whole body sees LI-4 combined with TE-5. Gallbladder points such as GB-20 and GB-21 are also used when treating wind-related symptoms in musculoskeletal therapy (see page 112).

LI-4 also has a use to improve the immune system or 'supplement the defensive qi'. It is normally used with LU-7 and ST-36 for this purpose, ST-36 to strengthen the stomach and aid in the generation of more qi, LU-7 and LI-4 helping to spread the qi to the whole body surface. LI-4 is an essential point in the treatment of all conditions affecting the head and face, including headache and neuralgia.

LI-11 is an essential point for clearing excess yang or heat (hence its use in shoulder pain) and may be combined with SP-9 to clear damp heat. Combined with LI-4, LI-11 clears stagnation (useful in bi syndrome) in both the elbow and shoulder.

Stomach

The stomach is a yang meridian and is one of the few yang meridians used to treat internal organs. Through internal connections to the spleen and stomach the meridian effectively treats digestive disorders, abdominal pain/distension, constipation and diarrhoea. From the point of view of musculoskeletal pain, the stomach meridian is important for knee pain particularly (ST-35 being the lateral Xiyan point). The stomach meridian tends to concentrate yang and to control blood. It is therefore important in conditions involving blood heat such as nosebleeds and fevers, and also psychiatric conditions (so called spirit disorders) including anxiety and depression. It is said to calm the mind.

Of all the stomach points, ST-36 is the most important, and one of the most important points in the body. It is said to pull energy down and in (contrast this with LI-4 which moves energy up and out) and is an important point for general supplementation. ST-36 draws energy into the stomach organ enabling it to more effectively extract nutrients. It is the most important point for epigastric pain of any sort.

The single most important point for transforming phlegm is ST-40. It may be combined with lung points (LU-9 or LU-5) in chest conditions and with SP-9 or SP-6 for general damp/oedematous conditions. The spleen's function of 'transformation' is said to be impaired in damp conditions and as the stomach and spleen are linked meridians, the use of ST-40 (luo-connecting point) with spleen points makes sense. ST-38 (one finger-breadth medial to ST-40) is an important distal point for frozen shoulder. ST-41 is an important local point in ankle conditions, especially arthritis.

ST-44 is used principally to clear heat from the upper reaches of the stomach channel, tending to drain it downwards and cool it. Examples of this include toothache, eye pain, and frontal headaches. ST-44 is often combined with LI-4 when treating these conditions.

Spleen

The spleen channel is chiefly used to treat dampness and lower limb swelling in cases of musculoskeletal pain. Conditions such as stiffness (fixed bi syndrome) affecting the knee, medial ankle and big toe are especially involved. In general acupuncture treatment the spleen also has uses in the treatment of gynaecological disorders and abdominal pain. SP-4 (luo-connecting point and confluent point) is most commonly used to link with the penetrating vessel (chong mai) to treat blood stasis including menstrual disorders, abdominal pain and fullness in the chest. SP-6 is the intersection point for the three yin meridians and is used extensively in gynaecological conditions. It is often combined with points such as LR-3, KI-3 and ST-36. SP-6 is important in the treatment of lower abdominal and genital pain including hernia, and also for treating dampness in general. When used to treat dampness SP-6 may be combined with SP-9 to increase urination, or with ST-36 to transform dampness. SP-6 may be used to treat medial shin pain (shin splints) and medial ankle pain. In this latter case SP-5 may be used in addition as a local point. For arthritic pain over the ankle a line of points over the dorsum of the joint may be palpated and needled if tender. These are GB-40, ST-41, LR-4 and SP-5.

Heart

The heart meridian is mainly used clinically to treat 'spirit disorders' with HT-7 being the most important point from this point of view. The heart channel may also be used to treat headaches involving dizziness and chest symptoms. HT-7 (called spirit gate), the source point of the heart channel is used for treating insomnia and palpitations and is the most important point for 'calming the spirit'. HT-3 may occasionally be used as a local point in cases of elbow pain and also has uses when treating chest pain.

Small intestine

The small intestine and bladder meridians are major yang ('Tai Yang') channels. This means that they are the outermost of the yang channels. As yang itself is exterior, this makes them energetically the most external channels and both give symptoms which are almost entirely external in nature, the organ systems rarely being affected. In the case of the small intestine, where organ symptoms are present the large intestine and Triple Energiser meridians should be addressed first, as the result is likely to be better. The small intestine is most commonly involved in local pain to the posterior aspect of the shoulder, with SI-9/10/11/12 being used as local points and trigger point for the rotator cuff muscles.

The most frequently selected small intestine point is SI-3 (tonification point). It is a commonly used distal point for occipital headache and for pain in the neck in general. The point is also used for fever when neck pain occurs as one of the symptoms and traditionally it is the 'malaria point'. In addition, SI-3 is an important local point for arthritic pain in the fingers. SI-8 may be used as a local point for posterior elbow pain such as olecranon bursitis or 'thrower's arm'.

Bladder

The bladder is the longest and widest of all the channels, and as with the small intestine it gives almost exclusively external symptoms. Local points along the bladder meridian should be palpated and needled if tender. Pain can occur anywhere from the head and eyes, through the whole spine and down the leg to the little toe. For the treatment of back pain BL-40 is one of the most important points, and is termed the 'command point' of the back. This point is said to release pathogens lodged in the joints along the bladder meridian. For this reason BL-40 may be used to treat pain in the posterior knee or hip. BL-57 (heavenly star point) is often used for lumbar pain with referral into the calf. Equally it is used for calf pain and cramps at night. The blood is said to return to the liver at night during sleep. If the 'liver blood' is deficient it is unable to nourish and 'soften' the calf muscles, hence the night cramps. The point is also a primary point in the treatment of haemorrhoids (the bladder-divergent channel winds around the anus). BL-60 is frequently selected for headache and neck pain as well as for lumbar pain. It is said to induce labour and is used to assist in difficult delivery. The point is therefore contraindicated in pregnancy.

BL-62 (confluence point) is used in the treatment of 'wind conditions' including headache. It may also be used as a local point for lateral ankle pain and for lumbar pain referred into the outside of the foot. When used for its function as a confluence point it is coupled with SI-3 to open and regulate the yang motility vessel.

Kidney

The kidney meridian treats the kidney organ as it is described in TCM. From the point of view of musculoskeletal pain by far the most important function of the kidney is that it 'dominates the bones'. It is used most often to treat chronic low back pain; the kidney-divergent channel travelling through the lumbar spine en route to the neck, where it converges with the bladder channel. The effect of bone dominance also makes the channel useful when treating chronic knee pain, especially when it is arthritic in nature. The kidney is the channel with the deepest energy level and the kidney organ stores the essence. The meridian is therefore associated with chronic illness in the elderly.

The position of KI-1 on the sole of the foot makes it too painful to needle, although direct acupressure is often extremely soothing. An alternative point is used if needling is required, and for electro-measurement, at the medial nail point of the 5th toe. KI-3 (source point) is normally needled in cases of kidney deficiency. The point may be used for general conditions such as sleeplessness due to yin deficiency (yang alternates to yin at night, if this switch fails to occur sleeplessness results), tinnitus (the kidney 'opens to the ear'), and sore throat (heat affecting the divergent channel). In the elderly the point is important as a 'root cause' in cases of chronic lumbar pain, and may be through-needled to BL-60. KI-5 is called 'water spring' and may be used to promote urination due to qi stagnation, common after surgery. For this purpose it is often combined with SP-6. The point is also used for menstrual disorders. KI-6 has a variety of general indications due to its function as a confluence point of the yin motility vessel. In musculoskeletal therapy KI-6 is used as a local point for treatment of the medial ligament of the ankle. The name of KI-7 (tonification point) is 'returning the flow' and reflects its use as a diuretic point. It is used to control swelling, especially lower body swelling, (often with SP-9) by tonifying the kidneys. It is also said to control sweating, where it is combined with LI-4. In musculoskeletal therapy KI-7 may be substituted for KI-3 in cases of chronic low back pain, if it is found to give a better deqi sensation. KI-10 is almost exclusively used as a local point for medial knee pain, especially if it is associated with hamstring bursitis, the point lying between the tendons of semimembranosus and semitendinosus.

Pericardium

The pericardium meridian is used clinically to treat many heart disorders. This is because the pericardium protects the heart and will combat a pathogen attacking the heart. If a pathogen does reach the heart the condition is very serious. In addition pericardium points are often used to treat stomach disorders and general pain in the upper abdomen such as heartburn. This has led some authors to refer to the pericardium channel as the 'stomach meridian of the arm' (Pirog, 1996). The pericardium is associated with the production of phlegm in TCM, and phlegm affecting the heart (the heart is said to 'house the mind') and is generally involved with psychiatric conditions including schizophrenia and epilepsy. In musculoskeletal treatment the pericardium is used to treat chest and rib pain, palpitations, and sub-axillary pain and swelling. PC-3 is used as a local point for medial elbow pain, and is often described as a similar point to BL-40, both of which are used to clear heat. PC-3 (and HT-3) is also used to reduce tremors in the head, arm, and hand.

PC-6 is the most popular point of the pericardium meridian. It is used mainly to reduce nausea (counterflow qi in the stomach in TCM terms), especially after surgery and is the classic antiemetic point (Dundee et al., 1989). Where nausea is associated with epigastric pain (heartburn or indigestion, for example), PC-6 may be combined with ST-36. Additionally PC-6 may be used with HT-7 to treat 'spirit disorders' such as anxiety, restlessness and insomnia. PC-7, which is located at the wrist crease between the tendons of palmaris longus and flexor carpi radialis, is used in the treatment of carpal tunnel syndrome. The needle is inserted obliquely to travel along the length of the carpal tunnel and passes beneath the flexor retinaculum (see page 186). PC-8 is analogous to KI-1 in the sole of the foot. Both are generally thought to be too painful to needle but may be used in acupressure. In addition both are used during the practice of qi gong to visualise energy passing into and out of the body. PC-9 is used clinically at the tip of the middle finger rather than at the radial nail point. This position is said to make it the most distal (and therefore powerful) of the jing well points. In addition, when the arms are raised above the head this point is the highest point of the body and therefore the closest to heaven. It is used to restore consciousness by pricking it rather than needling.

Triple Energiser

The Triple Energiser is said to be the second most superficial meridian and so especially susceptible to external pathogens. It is most commonly used in musculoskeletal therapy to treat lateral shoulder and neck pain, especially neck pain exacerbated by rotation (along with gallbladder points). The course of the meridian is around the ear and so it is also used to treat ear conditions such as deafness and tinnitus, along with kidney points as the kidney 'opens to the ear'. Triple Energiser points are indicated more for low-pitched tinnitus, which is said to be due to a pathogen, and occurs through sudden onset. This type is due to *excess* and made worse by stress and emotional factors. Kidney points are used more for high-pitched tinnitus, which is more chronic in nature, due to *deficiency*. This type is brought on through a slow onset and (because of the kidney involvement) often occurs with back or knee pain. Finally the Triple Energiser is used to treat headaches, especially those associated with the temples and sides of the head.

TE-2 and TE-3 are both used as local points for treating arthritis of the fingers. TE-4 (source point) due to its location on the dorsal wrist crease may be used for wrist pain due to arthritis or ligamentous sprain, either through shallow oblique needling or moxibustion. In addition, as the source point it may be used to build qi in the meridian. TE-5 (luo-connecting point and confluence point) is considered clinically the most important distal point of the meridian. The name of the point, 'outer pass' indicates one of its important uses, which is to draw energy out from the meridian if it is lodged through stagnation. The point is used especially for wandering-bi syndrome which is due to pathogenic wind, where it is often combined with LI-4. When used as a distal point for lateral shoulder pain it is combined with points such as TE-14 and GB-21. The point is a commonly used distal point for hearing disorders such as tinnitus and is often combined with gallbladder (GB-43) and kidney (KI-3) points for this purpose.

TE-10 may be used as a local point for posterior arm pain, lying as it does directly over the olecranon bursa, while TE-14 is an important local point for shoulder pain where it is normally combined with LI-15. TE-16 (as with SI-16, LI-18 and ST-9) may be palpated, and if painful used as a local point for the treatment of torticollis due to its proximity to the sternomastoid muscle.

Gallbladder

The gallbladder channel is implicated with pain in the eyes and ears, and lateral pain of the head, neck, trunk, and lower limb. It is especially important in cases of hip pain and low back pain referred into the lateral aspect of the leg. GB-2 (as with TE-21 and SI-19) may be used in the treatment of deafness and tinnitus due to its proximity to the ear. GB-14 is used in cases of frontal headache where it may be combined with LI-4 and ST-41. GB-20 is an important point to eliminate wind (often used with LI-11 and LI-4) and an important local point for neck pain localised to the occiput. GB-21 is used for neck pain extending into the trapezius, and as the meeting point of the gallbladder, Triple Energiser, stomach and yang linking vessel has a powerful action on the yang channels in general.

GB-30 (heavenly star point) is vital in the treatment of hip pain and low back pain referred into the hip. GB-31 may be used in cases of hip pain referred along the lateral aspect of the femur towards the knee. Its name 'wind market' implies its importance in the treatment of wandering-bi syndrome affecting the hip. GB-34 (influential point for sinews) is one of the most commonly used gallbladder points, selected in most cases of musculoskeletal pain, especially those which occur at multiple sites throughout the body. GB-37 (named 'bright light') is the luo-connecting point of the gallbladder channel and an important distal point for the treatment of eye disorders, where it is often combined with LR-3 (the liver 'opens to the eye').

GB-39 (influential point for marrow) is opposite SP-6 and is the crossing point for the three yang meridians (SP-6 being the crossing point of the three yin meridians). It is used in cases of lateral leg pain often in association with GB-30 and GB-34, and may be used in cases of chronic lateral neck pain where it is combined with GB-20 and TE-5, for example. GB-40 (source point) may be used as a local point for lateral ankle pain, and to energise the whole meridian if required. GB-41 and GB-43 may be selected as distal points for pain along the course of the gallbladder channel such as lateral head, neck, or trunk pain.

Liver

The liver channel is used for a variety of general conditions such as frontal headaches and pain around the eyes (the liver opens to the eyes), gynaecological disorders (the liver stores blood), and hernia (the liver channel enters the body at the inguinal region). In terms of musculoskeletal treatment, the liver is associated with medial knee pain and the contractile function of the muscles (the liver 'controls the tendons'). LR-3 (source point and heavenly star point) is the most commonly used point of this meridian. It is one of the 'four gates' points along with LI-4. It is used with general conditions such as headache, insomnia, and menstrual disorders, as well as musculoskeletal disorders such as lateral chest pain and lumbar pain radiating into the abdomen. The liver 'maintains the free flow of qi' and so in cases of qi stagnation, LR-3 is used. Stagnation may occur particularly with suppressed emotions such as anger. Since tumours and lumps in general are a result of stagnation, this point may be used in these cases.

LR-3 is said to 'subdue liver yang' and 'pacify liver wind'. The liver 'governs uprising' and where yang and wind rise upwards unchecked, headache and dizziness will result. This point is therefore essential in headache of an excess nature, where it may be combined with GB-20, for example. Because the liver 'controls the tendons' LR-3 may be used to treat tremors and muscle spasms throughout the musculoskeletal system. In this respect its use is similar to GB-34.

LR-8 (tonification point) may be used to treat difficult urination and retention of urine together with spleen and kidney points. In addition, its position anterior to the tendons of semimembranosus and semitendinosus at the medial edge of the popliteal crease makes the point useful in cases of medial knee pain as an alternative to KI-10.

Conception vessel

Both the Conception (CV) and Governing (GV) channels are extraordinary channels. However, they differ from the other extraordinary channels (see page 42) in that they each have their own acupuncture points. The CV channel originates in the perineum (the uterus in the female) and passes up the front of the body to wind around the mouth and terminate in the eye. In general acupuncture practice the channel can be used to treat local disorders. Points below the umbilicus treat urinary-genital conditions, while points from CV-8 to CV-21 treat the intestines, stomach, lungs and chest. The lower abdominal points CV-4, CV-6 and CV-8 house the deepest energies in the body and form an area known as the *dantian*. These points can be used to tonify and nourish the body in general.

CV-3 is the front mu point of the bladder and the meeting point of the conception channel with the spleen, liver and kidney vessels. As such it is a major point for disorders of urination including cystitis and is often combined with SP-6 and LR-3 for this purpose. CV-6 is the 'Sea of Qi' and is used to tonify yang especially in conditions where the patient is very weak. CV-8 in the centre of the umbilicus is contraindicated to needling, but can be treated with moxibustion for abdominal pain and diarrhoea. CV-12 is the front mu point of the stomach and fu organs in general. It is important in gastric disorders including nausea and vomiting. CV-17 is the influential point of the respiratory system and is used in chest conditions especially asthma. CV-22 may be used in attacks of bronchial disorders but the needling technique for this point is highly specialised.

Governing vessel

The governing vessel passes through the spine to the brain. The lower points, GV-1 to GV-5 are used to treat disorders of the anus and rectum including haemorrhoids and prolapse. Many of the points may be used as local point for back pain, and some may be used to treat 'spirit disorders', that is psycho-emotional problems. GV-4 (gate of life), GV-14 (sea of qi) and GV-20 are perhaps the most important points in musculoskeletal therapy. GV-4 is used in the treatment of lumbar pain to tonify yang in chronic cases. It is chosen especially in the elderly where it may be used with BL-23 the back shu point of the kidney, for example. GV-14 is the meeting point of the governing vessel with the six yang channels. It has a powerful action on clearing heat from the body and is in fact one of the principle points to treat disorders of sweating. In musculoskeletal therapy it is used most often to benefit the upper spine. In cases of neck pain the needle is angled towards the painful side.

GV-20 is used for headache and as it is located at the apex of the head it is the highest and therefore most yang point on the body. It is therefore especially useful in treating dizziness and migraine due to uprising yang and wind, and in these cases it may be used with LI-4. GV-26 on the upper lip may be used as a resuscitation point to restore consciousness in fainting or needle shock for example. The point may be needled, but is probably better simply pressed firmly with the edge of the fingernail.

Principles of point selection and combination in musculoskeletal therapy

Points may be selected from three main sources, *local*, *adjacent* and *distal* (Table 6.2). Local points are those which are close to the painful region and may be painful to palpation. Almost all points are capable of relieving pain by activating the channel. As we saw in Chapter 4 pain is often the result of obstruction and stagnation of qi within a channel. Needling will encourage the flow of qi and help to resolve the stagnation. If qi is not flowing into an area due to an obstruction further along the channel a reinforcing technique is used in an attempt to 'pull' qi into the region. If pain is due to the build up of pressure of a pathogen, a reducing technique is used to allow the pathogen to escape. Local points may also form active trigger points showing a positive jump sign (see page 122).

Points adjacent to the area of pain may be used to treat pain resulting in a meridian passing through an area, or to treat a trigger point referring pain into an area. For example, needling an ahshi point over the greater trochanter is often effective at treating hip pain.

Points distal to the painful area are used if they are on meridians passing through this region. Any point on the meridian may be used but clearly some are more effective than others, and most are located below the elbows or knees. The source point is used to regulate the whole of the meridian and also to affect the Zang Fu organ to which the meridian relates. Tonification (mother) and Sedation (son) points are obviously used to increase or reduce the amount of energy in a meridian and its related organ. In addition pain created through an imbalance in the Zang Fu organs themselves will require needling of points related to the organ. For example, eye conditions may be a result of a disorder in the liver and so LR-3 may be chosen as a distal point. Clearly LR-3 (between the 1st and 2nd toes) is distal to the eye.

Table 6.2. Examples of local and distal point selection.

Body area	Distal points	Adjacent points	Local points
Forehead	LI-4, ST-44	GV-20	GB-14
Temple	TE-5, GB-41	GB-20	Taiyang, GB-8
Nape of neck	SI-3, BL-60	GV-14	BL-10
Eye	SI-6, LR-3	GB-16	BL-1
Nose	LU-7, ST-45	GV-23	LI-20
Mouth and cheek	LI-4, ST-41	SI-18	ST-4, ST-6
Ear	TE-3, GB-43	GB-20	GB-2, TE-17
Throat	LU-10, KI-6	BL-10	CV-23, SI-17
Chest	PC-6, ST-40	LU-1	CV-17
Costal region	TE-6, GB-34	LR-13	LR-14
Upper abdomen	PC-6, ST-36	ST-21	CV-12
Lower abdomen	SP-6, LR-8	ST-25	CV-4
Lumbar region	BL-40, SI-3	BL-32	BL-23, BL-25

(From Xinnong, 1999)

In musculoskeletal treatment it is often the case that yang meridians, on the outer aspect of the limb, are in excess and so proportionally the yin meridian on the inner aspect of the limbs are deficient (see page 57). In this case points are selected to sedate the yang meridian and to tonify (support) the yin. This is known as 'treating the symptoms and supporting the core'. For example when treating shoulder pain large intestine (yang) points may be chosen. The paired meridian to the large intestine is the lung (yin) and this may be supported by needling LU-9, the source point and tonification point of the lung channel.

Finally some distal points are chosen using a formula (symptomatic) approach, that is, the point has been identified as being effective with that condition over many centuries of clinical practice. Often the reason for this effect may not be obvious. An example would be the use of ST-38 in cases of frozen shoulder. Other formula points include the influential points, for example, GB-34 as the influential point of sinews or BL-11 as the influential point for bones.

When describing an acupuncture point prescription some points near the painful site should be used together with some along the meridian(s) passing through the painful area. Any symptomatic points relevant to the patient's conditions should also be considered. Where several symptoms may be linked in a pattern, the practitioner should try to determine the Zang Fu organ affected and needle relevant points to affect the organ (often the source point), in addition to local points, to target the pain.

Acupuncture treatment methods

Safe needling practice

The most common type of needle used during the treatment of musculoskeletal conditions are pre-sterilised disposable Filiform needles. These are of stainless steel construction nowadays although traditionally other metals such as gold and silver were used with additional claimed benefits. The needle consists of four parts. The needle tip is ground to a point. The needle body or shaft is the part which enters the body and so should not be touched, to maintain asepsis. The needle handle is either copper or stainless steel if webbed, or plastic. The handle joins the shaft at the root, the last part of the needle to touch the skin if the needle is inserted to its maximum depth. Needles are classified by their diameter or gauge. Needles normally vary from 26 (0.45 mm) to 34 (0.22 mm) gauge, and in length from 0.5 (15 mm) to 5.0 (125 mm) cun.

Prior to needle insertion, a skin inspection should be carried out. Any skin lesions should be noted (in writing on the treatment records) in case it is claimed that these were caused by needling at some later date. Each needle should be inspected for faults before usage. Bent or faulty needles should be discarded. The skin should be clean before needling. Swabbing is generally considered unnecessary unless the skin is exceptionally dirty (Campbell, 2000) but any obvious dirt should be removed with simple washing. The practitioner must wash his/her hands for each patient prior to needling. Any skin lesions on the practitioner's hands must be covered with a sterile adhesive plaster. The patient should be resting in a supported lying position, either prone, supine, inclined supine, or side lying. Sitting positions increase the risk of fainting.

Filiform needles are thin and flexible and will bend (and possibly break) if inserted into the skin in a haphazard fashion. Two methods of insertion are generally used, guide tubes and free insertion. With a guide tube, the needle comes inside a narrow plastic tube just shorter than the needle itself. When the needle with guide tube is placed on the skin surface over the acupuncture point, a small section of the needle handle (generally 2–3 mm) stands proud of the guide tube. The free end of the needle handle is gently but firmly struck with one finger to push the needle tip through the skin rapidly and therefore with the minimum of discomfort. Once the needle is inserted, the guide tube is removed and the needle pressed in further to the required depth. The needle shaft should not be touched, only the needle handle. When using long needles (over 3 cun) they will tend to flex. To prevent this the needle shaft may be bowed slightly from the handle.

Needles without guide tubes may be inserted directly using a rapid single-handed 'flicking' motion. Alternatively the practitioner may grip the needle shaft close to the skin using a sterile cotton wool pad or dressing. The needle is inserted again with a rapid flicking action to allow the tip to pass through the skin as quickly and painlessly as possible. The sterile pad is then moved up the needle shaft slightly and the needle is pushed to the required depth. The use of alcohol on cotton wool, or isopropyl alcohol swabs can lead to additional problems in some cases. Firstly the astringent nature of these substances can cause further discomfort and secondly some subjects may have a sensitivity to these substances.

Just as it is important to insert the needle through the skin rapidly and then press it to the required depth, needle withdrawal follows a similar pattern. The needle is slowly withdrawn through the muscle and subcutaneous layer and then rapidly pulled through the skin layer to lessen discomfort. If the skin around the acupuncture point is pressed with the thumb-nail prior to needling, less discomfort will be produced by needling itself and the patient is distracted. Traditionally it is said that this pressure moves the qi and blood away from the point temporarily (qi and blood is dispersed), and this prevents damage to the 'defensive qi'. Equally when the needle has been withdrawn, pressure over the point will act as a counter-irritant to minimise pain, but more importantly will stop bleeding and lessen any bruising over the point. To reduce the chance of needle stick injury this pressure should be provided using the tip of a cotton wool bud rather than the practitioner's finger.

Three angles of insertion are generally used, perpendicular, oblique and transverse. During perpendicular insertion the needle stands at 90° to the skin surface and offers the greatest depth of insertion. The needle is inserted to a specific depth (see Chapter 5) to avoid the risk of damage to major body structures, and to promote the feeling of 'deqi'. From a traditional perspective deeper needling is used for those with a strong body constitution such as adolescents. More shallow needling is used for infants and the elderly. Some schools of western acupuncture however argue that the needle only needs to break the surface of the skin for a wound to be made sufficient to create an electrical discharge which affects the acupuncture meridian (Society of Biophysical Medicine, 1985). For oblique insertion the needles form either a 45° angle to the skin surface or a 20° angle (transverse-oblique insertion). With horizontal insertion the skin is pinched up between two fingers of one hand to form a fold. The needle is inserted along the skin surface with the other hand, into the skin fold. When using both oblique and transverse insertion methods, the needle tip is inserted at the acupuncture point and the shaft angles towards or away from it. The shaft faces along the acupuncture meridian, and is said to 'reinforce' the point if it faces with the direction of the meridian flow and to 'reduce' if it faces away from the direction of meridian flow.

Needling sensation

When an acupuncture needle is inserted there may be slight discomfort as the needle passes through the skin into the subcutaneous tissue and muscle below. Once this has occurred another sensation is felt, known as sensory propagation along the channel or 'deqi'. This is a deep pressure sensation sometimes experienced as paraesthesia. In general deqi is greater in peripheral points than in those placed centrally. In western terms deqi is said to be pain referral along neural pathways. Deqi does not restrict itself to single dermatomes, nor does it follow nerve pathways exactly. It has been suggested that the phenomenon is due to nerve impulses travelling from the acupuncture point to the spinal cord and then from here up and down to several spinal segments via interneuronal networks (Stux and Pomeranz, 1998). The deqi sensation is thus seen as an illusion in much the same way as pain referred from a deep soft tissue structure. In traditional terms deqi is said to be the arrival of qi and is considered essential for obtaining a therapeutic effect (Xinnong, 1999). The deqi sensation is considered to show that the acupuncture point is having an effect on the meridian and through this on the Zang Fu organ itself. In general if deqi cannot be obtained, it is thought that the needle has not been inserted in the correct point and should be partially withdrawn and inserted at a different angle. The needle is kept in (retained) for approximately 15–20 minutes after deqi is felt. The time of needle retention may be varied to produce reinforcing or reducing effects, as detailed below.

A number of methods may be used to promote the deqi sensation. The needle may be rotated to and fro, the coiled handle scraped with the practitioner's fingernail, and the handle may be plucked or shaken. In addition the related meridian close to the acupuncture point may be gently massaged using a stroking or finger-kneading technique to encourage the movement of qi through the meridian. This later method is particularly useful where there is qi stagnation.

Reinforcing and reducing

The energy (qi) within a meridian may be reinforced (increased) or reduced (decreased) by using specific points (tonification and sedation points, see page 69) and by using specific needling methods at a single point. A variety of methods of reducing and reinforcing are used in traditional acupuncture (Table 7.1). The reader is directed to Xinnong (1999) for a full description. Manipulating the needle while it is at a specific depth, and varying the depth of insertion are the two most frequently used methods. The needle is inserted to the required depth and the needle is then rotated to and fro to 180° or less. Rotating in a single direction tends to 'wind up' the muscle fibres and can increase pain. Rotating gently and slowly with small amplitude movements provides a reinforcing technique while rotating quickly with larger amplitude movements is reducing.

Table 7.1. Methods of reinforcing and reducing.

Reinforcing	Reducing
Small amplitude movements with weak stimulation	Large amplitude movements with vigorous stimulation
Slow, forceful insertion with rapid withdrawal	Rapid insertion with slow forceful withdrawal
Insertion during inhalation	Insertion during exhalation
Needling against the meridian flow	Needling with the meridian flow
Thicker needles	Thinner needles
Brief retention of needles	Longer retention of needles

(after Stux and Pomeranz, 1998)

By varying needle insertion/withdrawal and retention a reinforcing or reducing effect may also be produced. Using slow heavy pressure to insert the needle and rapidly withdrawing it will produce a reinforcing effect. Rapid and light insertion followed by slow, heavy withdrawal produces a reducing effect. It is as though the needle is pressing more qi into the body to reinforce and dragging excess qi out from the body to reduce. If the needle is inserted as the patient breathes out and withdrawn as the patient breaths in, the reinforcing effect is emphasised. If the needle is inserted as the patient breathes in and withdrawn as they breathe out, the reducing effect is emphasised. More simplistically, asking the patient to breath out as the needle is inserted distracts them and is especially useful for a very nervous patient. Retaining the needle for longer periods (15–30 min) is said to reinforce, for shorter periods (10–15 min) is said to reduce.

Moxibustion and warm needling

An additional stimulus may be obtained by heating the needle (warm needling) or heating the acupuncture point itself (moxibustion). A species of chrysanthemum '*Artemisia vulgaris*' is used for moxibustion. Traditionally it is said that the heat (yang) can 'open the twelve regular meridians ... to expel cold and damp' (Xinnong, 1999). In addition to heat, it is also claimed that the acrid odour can itself travel through the meridian to regulate qi and blood and expel cold while the bitter nature of the smoke can resolve damp. Moxibustion thus involves a combination of the heat itself and the properties of the moxa herb, an important consideration when seeking artificial alternatives. Moxibustion expels cold which may itself have led to qi stagnation and also induces smooth flow of qi. It is also said that moxibustion can act as a preventive therapy with points such as ST-36, CV-4, CV-6, CV-12 and GV-4 being used.

Two methods of moxibustion are generally used, moxa cones and moxa sticks, both may be purchased ready-made nowadays but traditionally the practitioner would have made up his/her own. Moxa cones are placed on the skin over the acupuncture point. Traditionally the cones could also have been placed on salt (point CV-8, the umbilicus), or a slice of garlic or ginger (with holes punched through them) for additional therapeutic effects. The cones are ignited and removed when they have burnt down by roughly 2/3rd or when the patient feels intense heat.

Moxa sticks are used either directly over an acupuncture point or to warm an acupuncture needle which is already in place. The stick is held like a pencil with the tip gripped by the middle fingers. The 5th finger should rest on the patient's skin to ensure that the stick never moves too close to the patient. The patient is asked to report when the feeling of mild warmth increases to become uncomfortable (but not burning) at which point the stick is moved away from the skin for 1–2 seconds and then replaced to allow the heat to build up once more. This procedure is repeated rhythmically over a 30–90 second period, over each selected point, until a mild erythema is present. When warming an acupuncture needle with a moxa stick, the tip of the stick is placed next to the needle body and the heat is conducted into the patient's tissues. As an alternative a small amount of moxa wool may be wrapped around the metal handle of the needle and ignited. This method is less popular nowadays due to the risk of the moxa wool falling directly onto the patient's skin. Several ready-made moxa wool 'caps' are available which have a metal base. These fit directly onto the needle handle and reduce the risk of the moxa wool falling off.

Moxibustion has a number of contraindications. As it is a form of heat, it should not be used in the presence of fever or inflammation, both 'excess' conditions. Moxibustion should be used with caution on the face because of the thickness of the skin in this region, and on the head because of the chance of igniting the hair. As with needling, the abdominal region and lumbosacral area should not be used as a first choice in pregnancy. Distal points should be selected instead, excluding those shown in Table 7.4.

In a hospital department moxibustion has two disadvantages. Some patients will not tolerate the smell of smoke of the technique, and the smoke may activate roof-mounted smoke detectors. Smokeless moxa is available and the heat from it causes the same effect. It is said to be slightly less effective than standard moxa because of the claimed therapeutic benefits of the moxa smoke itself. Heat from an infra-red lamp may be used to warm the needles, and as with the use of moxibustion to instigate warm needling, the heat is conducted along the shaft of the needle and into the patient's tissues. The chemicals contained within the moxa wool are also available in a spray form, to be used after artificial heating of a point.

Electroacupuncture

In Chapter 4 we have discussed the processes involved in pain and the relief of pain through acupuncture. Briefly acupuncture stimulates Aδ

nerves in muscle. The Aδ nerves release enkephalin in the dorsal horn of the spinal cord to inhibit the activity of nociceptive impulses travelling into the dorsal horn via C fibres. In the cortex of the brain, the Aδ fibres send collateral fibres to the medulla releasing endorphins to begin a cascade effect known as descending inhibition which uses serotonin as a transmitter.

To reinforce this process, electric current may be applied to the body either through surface electrodes, for example, when using TENS (transcutaneous electrical nerve stimulation) or through acupuncture needles. When using electrodes, the voltage used must be sufficient to overcome the resistance offered by the skin. Using a current of 20 mA a voltage of 40 V is required to overcome a skin resistance of 2000 Ω (White, 1999). This is because Ohm's law states that current (A) is equal to voltage (V) divided by resistance (Ω). When using a needle placed through the skin into muscle, the skin resistance is less, somewhere in the region of 600 Ω. Now, a voltage of only 12 V is required assuming a current of 20 mA.

Typically in electroacupuncture (EA) stimulation a voltage of up to 20 V is used with a current of 10–50 mA. The frequency is either low (< 10 Hz), medium (up to 100 Hz) or high (above 100 Hz). As the needles pass into muscle, the patient feels a 'pounding' contraction, which should not be intense enough to be painful. A pulse width of at least 0.05 ms is required to depolarise nerves and above this level smaller intensities of current are needed as the pulse width is increased, because the current is obviously acting for a longer period. With pulse widths above 0.5 ms however, C fibre stimulation is likely to occur causing pain. A biphasic current (one which passes firstly in one direction and then the other) is generally used to avoid the remote possibility of ionisation occurring between the needle and body tissues and causing a burn.

The selection of frequency is important as it helps to determine the neural transmitter released by the body. Low frequency stimulation below 10 Hz releases β endorphin in the brain together with enkephalin and dynorphins in the spinal cord. High frequency stimulation at 200 Hz produces serotonin. Low frequency stimulation of 3 or 4 Hz is thought to mimic manual needle stimulation.

In addition to the standard contraindications and cautions given for acupuncture needling (page 132) the presence of a cardiac pacemaker is an important consideration with patients receiving EA. Electroacupuncture has been shown to interfere with a demand pacemaker (Fujiwara et al., 1980). As the intensity of EA increased, only spontaneous beats were seen as the pacemaker was suppressed by the electroacupuncture current. The muscle contraction caused by EA is also a consideration. Powerful contraction in the presence of deeply placed needles can cause the needles to bend or break. The EA intensity should be strong enough for the patient to perceive a comfortable pulsing but not so strong as to cause forcible muscle twitching.

Many of the principles underlying the application of EA will be familiar to those using other forms of electrotherapy apparatus. The apparatus should be checked before application and the technique explained and demonstrated to the patient. Points are needled and deqi obtained before the electrodes are connected to the needles. Needling to at least 1 cun is required to ensure that the weight of the connector does not cause the needle to move. Crocodile clips are traditionally used to connect the unit to the needles, and the needle handle (if metal) is used to fasten the clip rather than the shaft as the connector may slip down the polished shaft. The wires trailing from the clip should be fixed to the skin using light adhesive paper tape to remove the drag from the needle. Clips are connected to the needle and removed from the needle only when the intensity of the unit is set to zero. The intensity is increased gradually so that the patient feels a slight tingling sensation. This may need to be increased further as the patient gets used to the sensation. The intensity of stimulation should be increased and decreased gradually to avoid a sudden burst of current.

Trigger point acupuncture

The use of acupuncture to treat painful trigger points is an area where 'East meets West' and both TCM and western medicine can be seen to offer similar views. It is therefore an area of treatment which both practitioners and patients can readily accept, and may often serve as an initial introduction to acupuncture for both. In traditional Chinese acupuncture painful local points are called Ahshi ('that's it!', or 'oh yes!') points and the practitioner needles the most painful point to relieve pain. In western medicine, a myofascial trigger point is described as a highly sensitive local area which often lies within a taut band of muscle fibres. In general terms a trigger point (TrP) can cause pain in a muscle either at rest or especially when the muscle is placed on stretch. By being painful when the muscle is stretched, the TrP prevents the muscle from lengthening and functioning effectively and so may give rise to further pain which is ichaemic in nature. The spot tenderness that a TrP produces will increase to palpation, the pain getting more intense as the palpation pressure is increased. Importantly, the palpation gives rise to the pain which the patient is complaining of. Reproduction of the patient's pain being one of the main diagnostic criteria. In addition to pain, palpation may also detect a 'taut band', a term which describes a group of muscle fibres close to the TrP which has a rope-like consistency. The TrP lies along the length of the taut band and the band itself may give a transient contraction known as the 'twitch response' (Baldrey, 1998) or 'jump sign' when it is plucked like a guitar string. In addition fibrositic nodules may be detected. These nodules have been shown to contain a larger quantity of water retaining mucopolysaccharide than normal, which may impair the oxygen flow of the muscle and activate nociceptors (Awad, 1990).

Trigger points may also give indications of underlying imbalances in the meridians themselves. When a number of points are found, their course should be noted, to see if it makes up part of any acupuncture meridians. Pain at a point may often infer a blockage and treatment with meridian massage may also be of benefit to disperse the blockage and free the circulation (of qi, blood, and body fluids) in the area. Trigger points may be connected into strings of related points called myofascial chains (Headley, 1990; Seem, 1993), and these chains often correspond to meridian pathways themselves. This has led some authors to discuss the interesting possibility that acupuncture points and meridians represent areas which are predisposed to dysfunction concomitantly and therefore provide a means of imaging myofascial pain and dysfunction (Seem, 1993).

The patient will often brace him/herself against the pain of the trigger point creating a guarding pattern or 'holding pattern' (Seem, 1993). These holding patterns lead to dysfunction including stiffness and reduction in range of motion and muscle wasting.

A TrP itself may be either *active* or *latent*. A *latent* TrP does not cause pain at rest, but only when palpated. The muscle it is associated with may however still be shortened and restrict movement. An *active* TrP may cause both pain and tenderness at rest or when the muscle is stretched during daily activities. Palpation of the active TrP causes pain and referral of this pain in a pattern which mimics the patient's main symptoms. As previously mentioned, the tenderness found at the TrP can be increased by putting the muscle on stretch and re-palpating the point.

Three main hypotheses exist for the pathogenesis of a TrP (Barlos and Mak, 1999). Firstly, it is thought that when the muscle is loaded persistently (overuse) it becomes ischaemic and as a result its concentration of ATP is reduced. In turn this may lead to a loss of control of the calcium pump with the result that the muscle contracts. Secondly, the muscle spindle may become hyperactive through a reduction in its threshold. This causes the spindle to produce contraction through a stretch reflex during normal daily activities. Finally, the motor endplate of the muscle may release acetylcholine too readily, again leading to unnecessary muscle contraction.

Clinically the TrP may be outside the patient's perceived area of pain and so objective examination and palpation are prerequisites to effective treatment. TrPs often lie at the motor point of a muscle within the main muscle belly (e.g. upper trapezius), or along the free edge of the muscle (e.g. supraspinatus) or at the muscle insertion (e.g. anterior scalene). The TrP may either be needled directly with a rapid insertion to initiate a jump response (Barlos and Mak, 1999) or by inserting the needle superficially above the TrP (Baldrey, 1998). As the needle is manipulated and the deqi phenomenon is felt, the patient may feel a replication of their pain pattern. To deactivate the TrP, the needle is left in place. In some cases superficial (5–10 mm) insertion and minimal (30 sec) stimulation is all that is required to deactivate the TrP. In other cases deeper needling and longer needle retention (20–30 min) may be required. Following treatment the TrP may be palpated once more to confirm that the point is no longer painful. The patient should be warned that occasionally needling will produce an exacerbation of symptoms for up to 24 hours before the pain then clears. In patients with acute pain and those with a fear of needling (so called 'strong reactors') a progressive approach is used, choosing shallow needling and short retention times initially. On retest, if some of the original pain is still present, deeper needling and longer retention times may be used. In general when needling a TrP, if the patient's referred pain and/or twitch response is reproduced, the likely outcome of treatment will be good, these two indicators having good prognostic value (Barlos and Mak, 1999). Following acupuncture treatment the muscle associated with the TrP should be stretched and gently but rhythmically contracted and relaxed. Exercise is a vital follow-up procedure to acupuncture in these patients.

Clinical note

When stretching a muscle associated with a TrP hold relax and/or contract relax procedures are used. Hold relax stretching involves taking the muscle to its end range and maintaining the position for 20–30 seconds. Tension in the muscle is registered by the Golgi tendon organ (a sensor in the tendon of the muscle) and autogenic inhibition results, causing the muscle tone to reduce. With contract relax stretching the muscle is stretched and held for 20–30 seconds. The muscle is then contracted isometrically against minimal resistance. When released, the muscle tone will reduce allowing the range of motion to be increased. Taking the upper fibres of trapezius as an example, a TrP is often located within the region of the acupuncture point GB-21. This is needled, and after the needle has been removed, the upper trapezius is stretched by combining shoulder depression with neck side flexion away from the painful area. Contract relax stretching may be performed by resisting shoulder elevation and neck side flexion towards the painful side.

Failure to follow acupuncture treatment with stretching and exercise to contract and relax the muscle may result in the TrP being re-established quite quickly. This is because pathological changes have taken place in the muscles as secondary effects to the TrP. These are the result of ischaemia largely and may include the formation of scar tissue. Gentle exercise to contract the muscle and stretch it will be required to regain the normal elasticity and muscle blood flow to the area and to re-establish the normal capillary bed.

Acupressure

Acupressure is the stimulation of acupuncture points and meridians using the fingers and hands rather than needles. It may be used where the use of needles is inappropriate such as in cases of needle phobia, but also enables the practitioner to incorporate acupuncture principles into more general treatment techniques such as physiotherapy. Three acupressure manipulations are generally used, point touch, point massage, and channel massage. In each case the intention is to balance energy within the meridian system. Point touch is performed by simply touching an acupuncture point with one finger, to transfer (balance) energy from one point to another or to draw excess energy from an area. It is claimed that each finger has either a positive or negative electromagnetic charge and that the right hand as a whole is positive and the left negative (Fig. 7.1). The middle fingers represent the polarity of the whole hand (right being positive, left negative). As electricity flows from negative to positive, to create a circuit from the patient through the therapist, the middle fingers are used on each hand (Cross, 2000). Deeper pressure is used to disperse energy and to release stagnation. The manipulation begins with light touch and builds up in a crescendo of pressure which the patient should experience as deep stimulation rather than sharp pain.

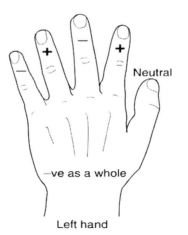 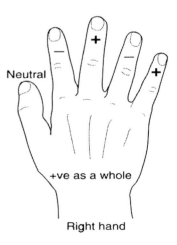

Figure 7.1. *Electromagnetic charges of the hands and fingers. (Reproduced with permission from Cross, 2000)*

Point massage may be used in chronic conditions to stimulate energy. A circular friction massage is used at and around the acupuncture point. Meridian massage may be used along the direction of energy flow to reinforce the meridian or in the direction opposite to the flow to sedate the meridian. Light pressure is used, and some authors claim that no skin contact at all is required to have an effect and the patient may remain clothed (Cross, 2000). Meridian massage is especially useful in chronic conditions to bring more energy into an area. For example, massage along the bladder meridian in cases of chronic low back pain.

Acute (excess) conditions should be sedated by placing the fingers on points above and below the lesion to enable energy to balance. Where profuse swelling and bruising is present, constant pressure is used beginning light and building in intensity to release the excess yang. Where this is too painful, some relief may be gained by selecting the same points on the opposite side of the body. A major point distal to the lesion should then be touched and held. A second point proximal to the point is then touched and the two held to balance the energy within the meridian. It is generally better (but not essential) to select two points on the same channel if this is possible.

Chronic (deficient) conditions are treated by stimulating distal points to summon/create energy by using point massage or deep pressure for as long as 2 minutes. A proximal point is then chosen to balance energy through the lesion. In addition to distal points and points along the meridian travelling through the lesion, influential points such as GB-34 (sinews) and BL-11 (bones) may be used. Command points (page 70) may also be used to great effect.

Periosteal acupuncture

Periosteal acupuncture is a technique where the periosteum covering the bone is needled directly by continuing the insertion depth until bone contact is made (Mann, 1992). The aim is to stimulate the richly innervated periosteum with either a single needle strike or multiple strikes, a technique referred to as 'periosteal pecking'. For this latter technique the needle is withdrawn slightly and reinserted at a slightly different angle to stimulate the periosteum above or below the initial site in a type of peppering pattern (Fig. 7.3). The pecking technique is used as a needle manipulation rather than twisting because the periosteum is too thin for twisting to 'wind it up', as is the case with muscle fibres for normal needle insertion. The sensation achieved with periosteal acupuncture is a deep knawing bone pain. The stimulation may be used to affect pain throughout a particular scleratome and does not seem to be point specific (Mann, 1992).

Periosteal acupuncture is particularly beneficial in areas where pain is located close to a superficial bony prominence. Examples include the common extensor origin of the elbow, the cervical articular pillars, the sacroiliac joint region and the occipital rim (Fig. 7.4).

(a)

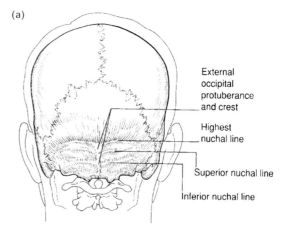

(b)

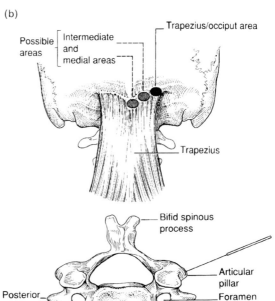

Figure 7.2. *Periosteal acupuncture points of the occiput and cervical spine*

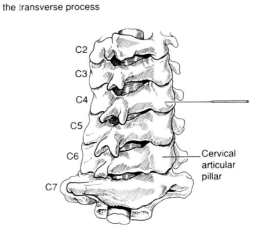

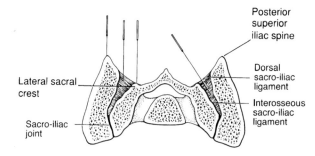

Adverse affects of acupuncture

A number of adverse affects of acupuncture have been reported (for a full review see Rampes and Peuker, 1999) and these are important for the lessens in prevention that they can teach.

Drowsiness and fainting

One of the positive effects of acupuncture treatment is its ability to relax the patient. This is especially important in cases where stress and/or anxiety forms an important component of the condition. Patients should always be warned of the likelihood of drowsiness following treatment in exactly the same way as they would when given medication. In addition it should be recommended that patients do not drive or operate machinery following acupuncture treatment until any drowsiness has worn off. Failure to draw a patient's attention to the potential dangers of drowsiness can result in severe consequences. Brattberg (1986) investigated the effect of drowsiness on patients ($N = 122$) receiving acupuncture in a pain clinic. Of this patient group 56 per cent were deemed to be a significant driving hazard had they driven home following treatment. Thirty-six per cent of the same group reported drowsiness with the risk of actually falling asleep, and 10 per cent actually slept following treatment. Although some patients get used to this effect, some may not. In the group above, 25 per cent still reported drowsiness after their third treatment, and importantly some

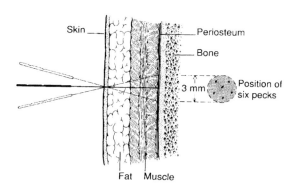

Figure 7.3. *Examples of sites for periosteal acupuncture. (Reproduced with permission from Mann, 1992)*

who had not experienced drowsiness during the first treatments later did so.

Drowsiness and fainting during treatment is an additional problem with acupuncture, and practitioners must be trained to know what actions to take should a faint occur. Needle fainting (syncope) usually occurs during the early stages of treatment before patients are accustomed to the treatment method. Fainting is more common in young males and in the elderly, and is more normally seen when patients are treated sitting upright. The incidence of syncope is small (less than 0.2 per cent) but significant (Chen et al., 1990). Convulsions following acupuncture treatment have also been reported (Hayhoe and Pitt, 1987) although whether the incidence of these complications is any greater than with other forms of treatment was not highlighted. To reduce the likelihood of needle fainting and the complications that this can bring, several actions may be taken (Table 7.2).

Table 7.2. Reducing the dangers of fainting during acupuncture treatment.

Explain the treatment to the patient before beginning.
Use supported lying positions to treat patients rather than sitting.
Never leave a patient unattended during acupuncture treatment.
Should fainting occur remove all needles and place the patient in the recovery
    position.

Infection

As with any invasive procedure, infection is always a potential risk with acupuncture. Certain steps may be taken to minimise this risk (Table 7.3) but the risk will always exist to some extent. Infection is more common when press needles or indwelling needles are used, especially with auricular acupuncture (Rampes and Peuker, 1999). Septicaemia has been reported following acupuncture (Doutsu et al., 1986) and in one case this resulted in intravascular coagulation of the knee joint (Izatt and Fairman, 1977). This later case is particularly relevant for the use of acupuncture treatment in musculoskeletal therapy of the knee using such points at Xiyan ('eyes of the knee') which enter the joint capsule. The same is true of the glenohumeral joint where points such as LI-14 and TE-14 may enter the joint capsule. Glenohumeral pyarthosis has been reported following acupuncture (Kirschenbaum and Rizzo, 1997).

Table 7.3. Reducing the risk of infection during acupuncture treatment.

Always use pre-sterilised, disposable needles.
Use each needle only once.
Never touch or handle the body of the needle.
Ensure that the patient's skin is clean prior to needling.
Ensure that the practitioner's hands are washed *prior* to treament.
Ensure that the practitioner's hands are washed *between* patients.
Be cautious about the use of press needles with patients who have prosthetic or
    damaged heart valves.

Endocarditis has been reported following acupuncture in patients with prosthetic heart valves (Jefferys et al., 1983), again following the use of press needles. This has led to the recommendation that patients with prosthetic or damaged heart valves not be given acupuncture involving the use of press needles (Rampes and Peuker, 1999).

The use of press needles in the ear (auricular acupuncture) is common in certain types of musculoskeletal acupuncture and for the treatment of obesity and smoking by lay practitioners especially. The practice of using press needles often involves the patient being recommended to touch or manipulate the press needle at regular intervals to 'maintain the effects of the treatment'. Unfortunately although pre-sterilised disposable press needles may be used covered with a sterile plaster, the plaster may fall off leaving the exposed needle to be manipulated in an open wound. Such needles are involved in almost all cases of perichondritis, and have been known to lead to permanent cosmetic deformity of the ear (Gilbert, 1987), the classic sportsman's 'cauliflower ear'.

Acupuncture has been shown to transmit hepatitis B (Slater et al., 1988). In all cases there was a lack of aseptic technique. Pre-sterilised needles had not been used and the needle tip had often been handled by the practitioner. It is interesting to note that a high incidence of hepatitis B exists in China where traditional Chinese acupuncture rarely relies on pre-sterilised needles. Lack of aseptic technique obviously endangers the practitioner as well, especially from needle stick injury. Removing the needles is a time when needle stick is particularly dangerous. A needle stick with a non-used pre-sterilised needle is not a serious problem. One with a needle which has been used on a patient most certainly is serious. The practice of using a single needle at multiple sites, removing a number of needles and gathering them in one hand, or of pressing on the needle hole with one finger leaves the practitioner open to the potential of needle stick with dirty needles. The recommendation must be to remove one needle at a time and place it in a sharps box before another is addressed. A single needle should be used at a single site only. If compression of the needle hole is required following treatment, a cotton bud should be used as it enables the practitioner to keep their hands well away from the withdrawing needle.

Trauma to body tissues

Injury to the heart/pericardium and lungs are amongst the most common complications of acupuncture with regard to direct trauma. In as many as 8 per cent of the population, foramen sternale exists where the central portion of the sternum fails to ossify during adolescence. This leaves only a thin membranous section beneath the skin covering the sternum and directly over the heart (Fig. 7.4). The average distance between the skin and the posterior surface of the sternum is 13–19 mm (Halvorsen et al., 1995). Use of the conception vessel points, especially CV-17, are most likely to cause heart injury where perpendicular needling is used rather than transverse. The abnormality cannot easily be found by X-ray but is identified using computerised tomography (CT) scan (Stark, 1985).

Pneumothorax may occur with perpendicular needling of acupunc-

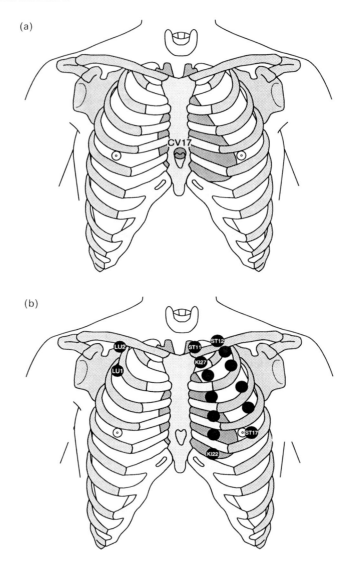

Figure 7.4. *Acupuncture points on the chest where deep needling may cause organ trauma. (a) Foramen sternales underlying CV-17. (b) Scheme of the chest ST-11–17; KI-22–27. (Reproduced with permission from Rampes and Peuker, 1999)*

ture points on the chest and those situated supra-clavicularly. In Japan, of more than 650 cases of pneumothorax, 9 per cent had been caused by acupuncture (Nakamura et al., 1986). A questionnaire about complications of acupuncture given to 1300 acupuncture practitioners and doctors revealed 33 cases of pneumothorax in total (Norheim and Fonnebo, 1995). The diagnosis of pneumothorax may be missed, and repeat X-rays may be required. The patient may complain of pain and a burning sensation in the chest and become short of breath. Needles inserted below a depth of 10–20 mm in the mid-clavicular line (stomach meridian), para-sternally (kidney meridian) or infra-sternally (lung meridian), depending on the subjects body build, risk reaching the pleura. In the medial scapular line (outer bladder meridian) the depth is 15–20 mm. Importantly, when needles are inserted it must be remembered that soft tissue compression occurs, so the insertion depth may be greater than the total needle length used.

Vascular lesions may also occur. It is fairly common for acupuncture points to bleed following treatment. In such cases a single drop of blood may be apparent and in some approaches this may be desirable (Xinnong, 1999). However, several points lie directly over superficial arteries and more serious vascular damage may result from inappropriate deep needling. The point BL-40 located in the centre of the popliteal fossa lies directly over the popliteal artery, for example, and oblique needling to a maximum needle depth of 1 cun is normally recommended. Perpendicular needling with longer needles runs the risk of arterial damage.

Trauma to the spinal cord may occur when needling governor vessel points or inner bladder line points especially. The depth of the spinal cord varies from 25–45 mm depending on body build so oblique needling to a depth of no more than 1.0–1.5 cun would seem sensible. The use of needle retention, less common in the west, gives the additional risk of needle migration or needle movement from the patient falling. Retention of needles is not to be generally recommended due to the likelihood of needle migration. Injury to peripheral nerves such as the medial nerve within the carpal tunnel (PC-7) or the fibular nerve close to the head of the fibula (GB-34) may also occur causing paraesthesia or, unusually, long-term injury.

Management of acupuncture incidents

A number of possible incidents may be encountered in the day to day use of acupuncture as with any therapeutic intervention. The practitioner should use his/her basic first aid knowledge augmented with some special considerations characteristic of acupuncture. All incidents, however minor they may seem at the time, should be recorded, in detail, in writing. Record exactly what happened in terms of therapy, what was done to prevent the incident, and what actions were taken as a result of the incident. If a witness is present they should also be asked to record the actions taken.

Fainting

Overall management of fainting is the same as at any other time, with the obvious difference that needles are present. If a patient feels drowsy and faints, the first action must be to remove all of the acupuncture needles. The patient should then be moved into the standard recovery position and given plenty of fresh air. Any restrictive clothing should be loosened and needling should not be re-started in the same treatment session. The point GV-26 on the upper lip may be used to aid resuscitation. Deep pressure should be used on the point using the practitioner's fingernail for 30 seconds.

Stuck needle

A needle may become stuck through muscle spasm. In addition if the needle has been manipulated with rotation in a single direction (rather than to and fro) the muscle fibres may bind the needle instigating spasm as well. The patient should be encouraged to relax and the needle manipulated very gently to see if it can be coaxed to move. If unidirectional rotation has caused it to stick, use rotation in the opposite direction. Gently massage the skin area around the needle aiming to press the skin down away from the needle to release it. Sometimes placing another needle by the side of the first will reduce spasm and release the first.

Bent needle

Each needle should be inspected before insertion to avoid inserting a needle which is bent. On insertion the needle may bend if it is pressed in too hard, or if it strikes bone. By far the most common cause of a bent needle however is the patient moving during the retention period. The needle becomes difficult to rotate, and to withdraw directly. Stop manipulating the needle and withdraw it slowly, following the bend of the needle. It may take several minutes to completely withdraw the needle, pulling a little at a time.

Broken needle

A broken needle is a far more serious situation and it is vital that the practitioner is sure that all of the needle has been removed. With the advent of pre-sterilised disposable needles the quality of needles has been improved, and luckily needle breakage is far less common. However, it can still occur through insertion or manipulation which is too forceful, or if the patient moves when the needles are in place. The weakest portion of the needle is generally the point at which the handle joins the shaft. For this reason a needle should never be inserted completely to the end of the shaft, a small amount of the shaft as well as the handle should always remain above the skin.

If a broken needle occurs, the patient should not move as this will encourage the needle to move further inwards. If a small portion of the needle is visible above the skin, this part should be gripped with tweezers and the needle removed. If the broken end of the needle lies flush with the skin, the surrounding skin may be gently pressed down below the level of the needle end to enable it to be gripped with tweezers and again removed. When the needle has gone too deep to be removed by hand, it will require surgical removal. The patient must be escorted to hospital without moving the limb which contains the needle. The practitioner should take other needles of the same type and size for use as reference for hospital staff.

Contraindications

Several contraindications exist to acupuncture (Table 7.4). Needling of the top of the skull is forbidden in infants as the fontanel has not yet closed. Lower abdominal points and the lumbosacral region should be needled with caution in pregnant females. The points LI-4, SP-6, BL-67 and BL-60 are contraindicated during pregnancy as they are used to facilitate childbirth and may lead to miscarriage. Because of the risk of miscarriage and any litigation effects the lower abdomen and lumbosacral region should not be needled during the first three months of pregnancy. After the first three months of pregnancy, points on the upper and lower abdomen and lumbosacral regions should not be needled. Distal points should be used instead.

Table 7.4. Contraindications and cautions to acupuncture.

During pregnancy points LI-4, SP-6, BL-67, BL-60.
During the first trimester (three months) of pregnancy points on the lower abdomen and lumbosacral region (caution).
After the first trimester of pregnancy points on the upper and lower abdomen and lumbosacral region (caution).
Patients with haemophilia.
Epileptic patients who have had a fit during the last three months.
Diabetes?
Prosthetic and damaged cardiac valves (no press needles).
Pacemaker (no electroacupuncture).
Metal sensitivity or allergy.

(Rampes, 1998; Rampes and Peuker, 1999)

Fearful patients should not be needled, moxibustion or acupressure may be used instead. Nervous patients should be needled only using points which they cannot see.

Patients with haemophilia should not be needled as there is a risk of internal bleeding, and epileptics should not be needled if they have had a fit in the last three months and then few needles should be used. In general it is better to use as few needles as possible to obtain the required therapeutic effect.

Patients with diabetes should be treated with caution. In traditional Chinese acupuncture an extra point exists to treat diabetes (in TCM called 'wasting and thirsting disorder'). Known as *Weiguanxiashu* it is the stomach controller lower shu point and lies 1.5 cun lateral to the eighth thoracic vertebra (T8), on the inner bladder line between BL-17 and BL-18. The loss of peripheral circulation, and reduced skin sensation and healing rate that diabetics may suffer, makes the use of points on the hands and feet especially dangerous. Certainly the use of any kind of heat including moxibustion is contraindicated, and peripheral points must be used with extreme caution. Acupuncture may alter blood sugar levels (Hopwood et al., 1997) and patients should be warned to monitor this, as a hypoglycaemic destabilisation may occur.

Lower limb treatment protocols

Introduction

The treatment protocols given in the next three chapters draw on both western and TCM acupuncture principles. From a western perspective pain relief is often the dominant requirement and local (ahshi) points and trigger points referring into the painful area are used. From a TCM viewpoint, channel obstruction which may cause qi stagnation or deficiency/excess must also be considered. Distal points are therefore selected for their ability to treat the underlying imbalance which may exist in parallel with the pain.

It is said that yang has a tendency to excess and yin has a tendency to deficiency. Where pain is experienced on the yang aspect of the limb, points along the affected meridian are therefore chosen and will often be sufficient to relieve pain. For a more effective long-term result however, supporting the yin meridian internally/externally related to the affected yang channel is required. This is why at times points seemingly unrelated to the pain are selected. It should also be noted that by needling both meridians of an internally/externally linked pair the flow of qi is increased and stagnation more effectively removed. In cases of pain along a yin meridian, deficiency often underlies the pain (for example, chronic arthritis). Local points may again be chosen together with distal points on the affected meridian. However, to bring qi into the channel, the luo-connecting points may be required and other points designed to support the body system in general, such as influential points or points to support qi or blood may be used.

When the symptoms suggest that both the yang and yin meridians are affected and pain is on both sides of a limb, or symptoms of two Zang Fu organs exist, source points and luo-connecting points may both be used. In general the source point of the more affected meridian (the 'host') is used together with the luo-connecting point of the less affected meridian (the 'guest'). This approach is sometimes called guest–host treatment (Ellis et al., 1994).

This type of approach treats a musculoskeletal condition on three levels, basic, system and symptom (Society of Biophysical Medicine, 1985). The *symptom* level addresses tender points which when needled reduce pain. These points are ahshi points in TCM, Kori points in Japanese acupuncture or trigger points in western acupuncture. The *system* level addresses the acupuncture meridians travelling through the painful area both yin and yang. Distal points on the same or coupled meridians are therefore used. *Basic* (core) level treatment addresses fundamental energy imbalances which underly the musculoskeletal condition and may be seen as the 'cause' of the condition. For example, an external pathogen (cold, damp or wind) may attack the body surface but only penetrate if the body's defensive qi has been weakened. The term 'cause' has many meanings of course. In western medicine the 'cause' of knee pain may be arthritis (the medical diagnosis). In terms of meridian acupuncture the 'cause' of the knee pain may be a combination of cold, wind and damp invading the channels (the invading pathogen). Alternatively the 'cause' may be said to be the underlying deficiency which failed to make the body strong enough to resist the invasion (the body imbalance).

Although a patient with a musculoskeletal condition comes to see a practitioner primarily for the relief of their symptoms, (pain, stiffness, pins and needles, for example), a treatment can only be truly effective if a more in-depth holistic (whole person) approach is taken.

Protocols

Full assessment of the patient must be made taking into account questions and tests relevant to both western medicine and TCM. Of particular note is pain referral from the lumbar spine or hip into the leg. Neurological examinations such as the slump test (see Norris, 1998) will readily differentiate between local pain and referred pain, and is dealt with below.

The foot

Metatarsalgia

Metatarsalgia occurs when the transverse arch of the foot flattens. Ordinarily the transverse arch is supported by the peroneus longus muscle which pulls the medial and lateral edges of the foot together. Distally the transverse arch is formed by the metatarsal heads and more proximally by the cuneiform bones. Flattening of the arch allows the metatarsal heads to descend, bringing the central heads into greater contact with the ground. Pain typically occurs to the 2nd and 3rd metatarsal heads after prolonged standing and walking on hard unforgiving surfaces. The 2nd metatarsal head should be the highest point of the arch forming a 'keystone'. In walking, the metatarsal heads contact the ground with the greatest amount of force being taken by the 1st metatarsal phalangeal joint. The arch is held together

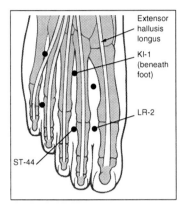

at the level of the metatarsal heads by the transverse metatarsal ligament and the contraction of adductor hallucis muscle during the mid-stance period of the gait cycle. In metatarsalgia the metatarsal heads splay apart due to a combination of poor foot musculature, prolonged usage, and often obesity.

Acupuncture treatment is aimed at relieving pain and is coupled with physical management using padding and taping to support the arch and rest the inflamed structures. Long-term management involves foot muscle restrengthening, footwear advice and often diet for weight loss.

Traditional acupuncture points in the area include LR-2 and ST-44 dorsally, and these may be needled if painful. These two points together with GB-43 form three of the four bafeng ('eight winds') points located 0.5 cun proximal to the web spaces of the toes on each foot. KI-1 on the sole of the foot may also be painful, but is more normally tender if metatarsalgia is combined with plantarfasciitis.

Needling ahshi points is of some benefit, but periosteal acupuncture directed at the metatarsal head is probably the treatment of choice. The needle may be inserted from the plantar surface of the foot directed to the metatarsal head until bone contact occurs. The most painful head is chosen (usually the 2nd) and the needle strikes the junction between the metatarsal head and the shaft. Pain over the lateral aspect of the transverse arch may be similarly treated using a periosteal technique over the 5th toe (Fig. 8.1).

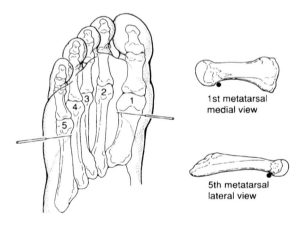

Figure 8.1. *Periosteal acupuncture in metatarsalgia. (Reproduced with permission from Mann, 1992)*

Mobilisation procedures together with taping are used in parallel with acupuncture. Traction and/or longitudinal mobilisation of the 2nd and 3rd metatarsal phalangeal joints is used. The foot is grasped in one hand, the toe in the other. A gentle and rhythmic oscillation is performed, trying to 'lengthen' the toe in its open pack (midway between flexion and extension) position. The patient will often find this relieves pain and may say that their foot often feels as if the toes need to be 'pulled'.

Padding is designed to lift the metatarsal heads away from the ground and may be supported with taping to assist this. A pad is shaped to clear the 1st metatarsal head and avoid placing excessive pressure on this joint, and to lift the central three metatarsal heads from the ground (Fig. 8.2). Zinc oxide (non-elastic) taping is placed around the forefoot to prevent the metatarsals from splaying when weight is taken through the foot.

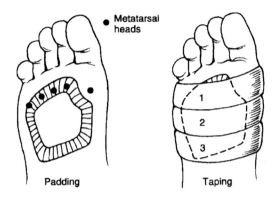

Figure 8.2. *Metatarsal padding and tape*

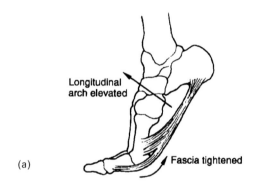

(a)

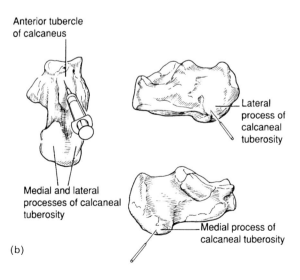

(b)

Figure 8.3. *(a) Plantarfascia action. Raising on to the toes tightens the plantarfascia and raises the longitudinal arch. (b) Plantarfascia treatment. (b has been reproduced with permission from Mann, 1992)*

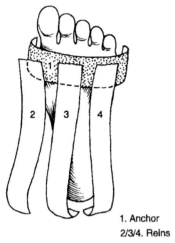

1. Anchor
2/3/4. Reins

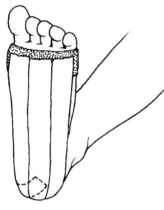

Figure 8.4. *Plantarfascia taping*

Plantarfasciitis

Plantarfasciitis is inflammation of the plantarfascia, a structure stretching from the medial tubercle of the calcaneus to the metatarsal heads. Overuse of this structure can cause inflammation at the fascial insertion in parallel with micro tearing. Pain is often felt as the patient pushes off from the toes lifting the heal. This is because when weight bearing, dorsiflexion causes the fascia to tighten and wind around the metatarsal heads and raise the longitudinal arch of the foot (the windlass effect) (Fig. 8.3a).

Acupuncture treatment is aimed at a periosteal point on the medial calcaneal tuberosity (Fig. 8.3b) The foot is treated with the ankle plantarflexed to relax the fascia. The patient lies prone with the knee flexed and the foot supported on a pillow. The needle passes through the relatively tough plantar skin and is angled towards the medial tubercle. Insertion stops when the needle strikes bone. Local pressure massage may also be used along the length of the plantarfascia and tenderness is often found over KI-1 in the sole of the foot.

Taping may be used to support the fascia on weight bearing. Non-elastic (zinc oxide) taping is used. The foot is placed in neutral position (between plantarflexion and dorsiflexion). An anchor is placed beneath the metatarsal heads and two or three strips (depending on the width of the foot) stretch from the metatarsal heads to the heel. The tape must pass over and behind the heal to prevent it slipping (Fig. 8.4).

First metatarsal phalangeal (MP) joint

The 1st MP joint has a fairly complex structure. The joint is reinforced over the plantar aspect by the plantar accessory ligament (volar plate), a strip of fibro cartilage formed from the transverse metatarsal ligament and the tendons of flexor hallucis brevis, adductor hallucis, and abductor hallucis. Two small sesamoid bones are formed within the ligament which serve to increase the weight-bearing area of the MP joint. A number of conditions can cause pain in the joint.

Turf toe is a traumatic injury which occurs in sport mainly, but is also seen in jobs which involve repeated kneeling, such as plumbing. Through forced extension of the MP joint the plantar aspect of the joint capsule is sprained and in some instances the sesamoid bones may be disrupted. Their collateral ligaments are damaged at the same time and the joint appears red, swollen, and painful. Bony alignment is normal.

In hallux limitus and hallux rigidus the 1st MP joint has reduced or obliterated movement. Pain is made worse when wearing shoes with a flimsy sole and better when wearing work boots, for example, with a stiff sole. Hallux valgus is a 1st MP condition where the joint is hyper-mobile and over time the joint deviates into adduction (and often axial rotation as well). Pain is through overstretch of soft tissues and degeneration of the joint itself. The condition is often worse in cold, damp weather (fixed bi syndrome, leading to bone bi syndrome see page 54).

Treatment of turf toe is aimed at pain relief using a reduction technique to drain excess yang. Local periosteal points around the 1st

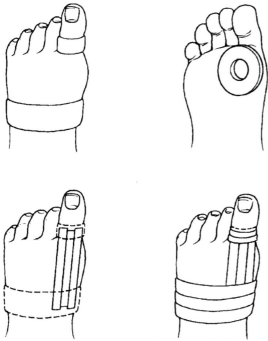

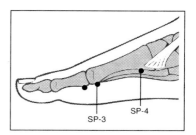

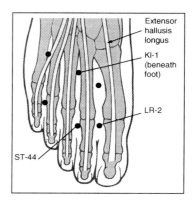

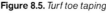

Figure 8.5. *Turf toe taping*

MP joint may be used together with LR-2 and SP-3. In cases of fixed bi syndrome SP-3 is especially useful as the source point of the spleen channel and for its ability to resolve dampness. SP-9 may be used as a distal point in cases of severe and/or chronic swelling. Cold or ice may be used in addition to reduce acute inflammation.

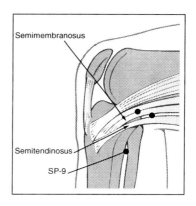

In sub-acute cases taping may be used to stabilise the 1st MP joint (Fig. 8.5). Anchor tapes are placed around the phalanx and mid-foot and then strips of non-elastic tape are placed across the dorsal and plantar aspect of the joint from the toe to the mid-foot. An oval piece of orthopaedic felt may be placed beneath the 1st MP joint to pad the area and reduce impact shock.

In cases of joint degeneration (hallux valgus and hallux rigidus) the same local points are used with the addition of GB-34 (influential point for sinews) and BL-11 (influential point for bones) on the same side as the painful joint. Moxibustion and warm needling of the local points is of use where pain is increased in cold/damp weather.

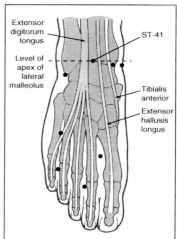

Mobilisation procedures are also important in cases of chronic joint degeneration. The therapist grips the forefoot with one hand and the 1st phalanx with the other. A rhythmic longitudinal oscillation may be used to mobilise the joint, or accessory movements gliding one bone upon the other with minimal movement. First MP joint abduction is useful in cases of hallux valgus especially.

In the elderly, painful obstruction syndrome may affect all the toes with particular localisation over the 1st MP joint. In this case heat and throbbing may be present in the toes and feet in general (especially at night) due to yin deficiency. Again local points may be used but distal points are also essential to strengthen the yin. ST-41 may be needled to affect all the toes, obtaining deqi travelling into the toes themselves. KI-3 may also be used to nourish yin and clear deficiency heat.

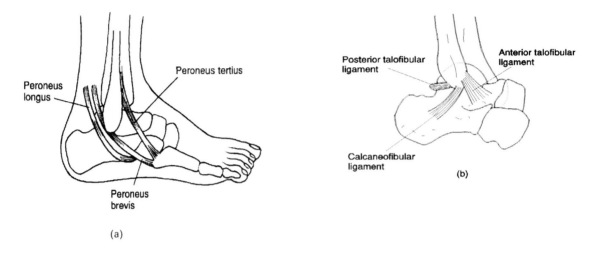

(a)

(b)

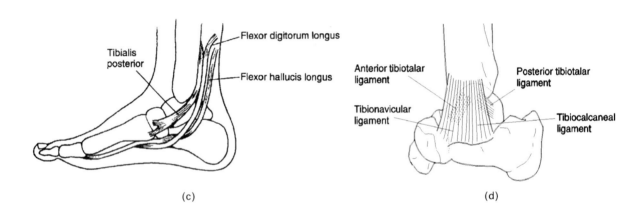

(c)

(d)

Figure 8.6. *Structures at the side of the ankle in relation to acupuncture points. Tendons near the malleoli, (**a**) lateral view, (**c**) medial view. Ankle ligaments, (**b**) lateral, (**d**)*

Ankle

Sprain

The most common traumatic soft tissue injury to the ankle is sprain to the anterior talofibular ligament, the anterior-most portion of the lateral collateral ligament itself. This structure (Fig. 8.6a) lies directly over GB-40 and this point is often used as a local point for treatment. The calcaneofibular ligament, the middle band of the lateral ligament may sometimes be involved, and again this structure is near an acupuncture point, this time BL-62. During forced inversion of the ankle, the movement which causes ligament sprain, the peronei muscles are often overstretched, with peroneus brevis attaching to the base of the 5th metatarsal the most usually affected muscle. The attachment of the peroneus brevis to the tuberosity on the base of the 5th metatarsal coincides with the points BL-63 (posterior to the tuberosity) and BL-64 (anterior and inferior to the tuberosity) and either may be needled if tender. Where redness, pain, and swelling are present a reducing technique is used.

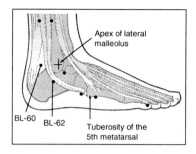

Physical therapy treatment includes taping to prevent further injury while allowing the inflammation to settle. The ankle is everted and dorsiflexed to shorten the overstretched ligament, and either strip or continuous taping may be used (Fig. 8.7). Exercise is then begun to restrengthen the ankle. Initially eversion movements are used against a resistance, such as elastic bands used in aerobics classes and physiotherapy, for example. As pain eases, weight-bearing (foot on the ground) exercise is begun to build the muscles up which hold the ankle firm (stabilise) and stop it 'giving way'. Simply standing on one (the injured) leg is enough to begin with. This can be progressed to standing on one leg and slowly twisting the upper body and then gently hopping and skipping. The aim is to develop the ankle to a point where it feels strong and secure even when walking or jogging on uneven surfaces.

Old ankle sprains often suffer from stagnation of qi and blood in the area, and acupuncture and/or acupressure may be used to remove stagnation. In addition to local points, distal points are used to encourage the flow of qi along the meridian. BL-60 (heavenly star point) is useful to clear heat and to activate the channel and so may be used in both the acute and chronic stages of ankle sprain, although obviously with a reducing method in acute injuries. GB-34 is particularly useful in chronic cases to activate the channel but also due to its action as the influential point for sinews.

Less usually the medial (deltoid) ligament may be affected (Fig. 8.6b). The local point for this structure is KI-6 for pain in the ligament itself or occasionally SP-5 for pain at the osseous junction of the ligament on the anterior aspect of the medial malleolus. Rehabilitation emphasising stability exercises in single leg standing are as important as for the lateral ligament following the resolution of pain.

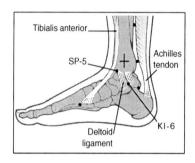

Arthritis

Arthritis may affect any of the joints of the foot and ankle, but it is more common in the weight-bearing joints including the subtalar and ankle joint itself. Arthritis usually occurs only after a history of fracture or repeated ligamentous injury leading to instability. In terms of TCM the patient often complains of a dull aching pain indicating a cold syndrome of the deficiency type and heaviness indicating damp, causing stagnation of blood and qi. Initially painful or fixed bi syndrome is present progressing to bone (chronic) bi with osteophytic lipping of the joint. Three points are useful in the treatment of this condition, SP-5, GB-40, and ST-41 as all three are positioned near the joint line. GB-40 is useful for lateral pain, SP-5 for medial pain and ST-41 for anterior pain. SP-5, in addition to being a local point will also dispel dampness. In some cases this point may be joined by through needling (beneath the tendons) to joint ST-41. Both ST-41 and SP-5 are jing-river points and it is said that external pathogenic factors are deviated towards bones and joints at these points (Maciocia, 1989). This makes them

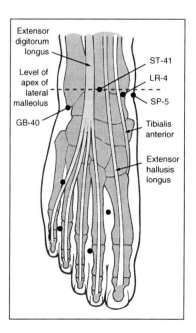

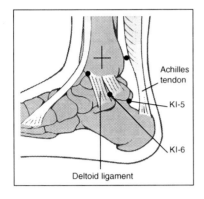

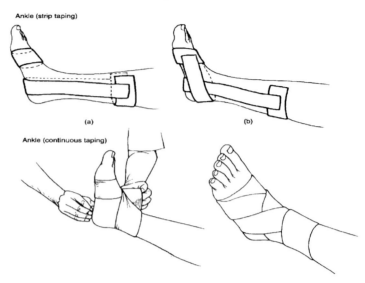

Figure 8.7. Ankle taping. (**a**) *Place elastic reins around the forefoot and mid-calf. Place the first stirrup from calf rein, and beneath the heel. Place a second stirrup from the forefoot rein around the calcaneum. Alternate stirrups building up a 'basket weave' taping. (**b**) Ankle (continuous taping). Evert and dorsiflex the foot (for an inversion injury). Begin the taping on the outer edge of the foot. Take it across the dorsum of the foot, and beneath the sole pulling the foot into eversion. Loop around the lower shin forming a figure of eight. Leave the heel free to enable the patient to wear a shoe*

Clinical note – Influential points

With a condition such as arthritis of the ankle or knee the question arises, which influential point should be used. BL-11 (bones), GB-34 (sinews) or GB-39 (marrow). GB-34 is used for stiffness and tightness of the muscles and joints in general, but especially for disorders of the knee and leg. GB-39, the influential point for marrow, focusses almost entirely on bone marrow, having little effect on the 'sea of marrow' (the brain) and is not often used to treat disease of the head and brain. It is mainly used for weakness, flaccidity, contraction and pain in the limbs. BL-11 is mainly used for bone diseases and rigidity of the spine as a whole and is less used for limb conditions.

---

particularly useful when treating ankle arthritis as they will act to release the pathogen. As with all cases of arthritis GB-34 or BL-11 may be used as distal points to influence sinews and bone, respectively. All three points may be used with warm needling.

Arthritis of the subtaloid joint (STJ) is a common condition which is often misdiagnosed. The patient usually has a history of a fall onto the heel but may simply be obese. Compression forces on the STJ are increased leading to inflammation and eventually joint degeneration. There may be osteophytic lipping. Pain is dull and gnawing in nature and exacerbated by cold/damp weather and prolonged weight bearing. It is made worse with hard footwear and correspondingly better with springy shoes. Acupuncture treatment aims at local painful points including periosteal points. Both KI-6 and KI-5 lie near the joint line of the STJ over the medial aspect which tends clinically to be the more painful side.

Joint mobilisation of the STJ is of benefit to try to regain some flexibility in the joint. Distraction techniques and localised movements are particularly useful. Gross movement of the STJ may be obtained by the practitioner cupping the heel in both hands (Fig. 8.8a) and performing forceful inversion and eversion by slowly swinging his/her hands and forearms from side to side in an arc. Distraction may be achieved by the practitioner gripping the lower leg with one hand and cupping the patient's heel in the other. The mobilisation force is either directly caudally in line with the tibia with the patient supine (Fig. 8.8b) or caudally in line with the foot with the patient lying prone (Fig. 8.8c).

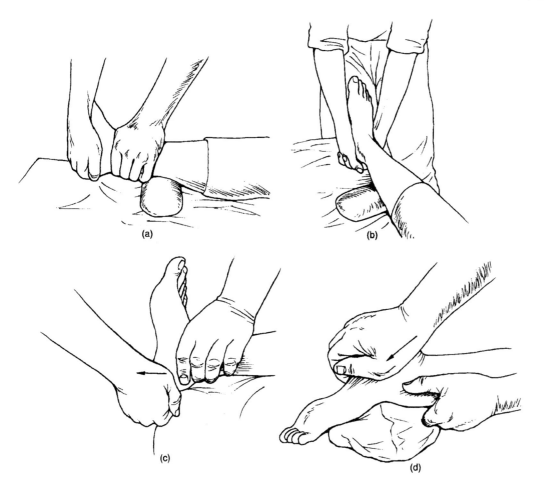

(a)

(b)

(c)

(d)

Figure 8.8. *Mobilisation of the subtaloid joint. (a) Stabilize lower leg and move talus. (b) Gross sub-talar movement. (c and d) Distraction and gliding*

Tendonitis

The tendons of peroneus longus and brevis pass around the lateral malleolus and those of the tibialis posterior, flexor digitorum longus and flexor hallucis longus pass around the medial malleolus (Fig. 8.6). Inflammation of the tendons (tendonitis) or inflammation of the tendon sheaths (tenosynovitis) may occur through repetitive movements such as jogging especially if footwear causes pressure over the area. The tendons may be thickened and painful with palpable crepitus occurring to repeated movements. In some cases the retinacula holding the tendons down may also be involved. As previously mentioned the peroneus brevis may be involved following the inversion forces involved during a lateral ankle sprain. In addition in sport, high levels of trauma can cause the tip of the lateral malleolus to become detached, allowing the peroneal tendons to dislocate during movement. This type of injury is usually the result of a forced dorsiflexion in activities such as soccer and skiing, for example. The flexor hallucis longus passes behind the medial malleolus and beneath the sustentaculum tali in a fibro-osseous tunnel which predisposes the tendon to mechanical irritation.

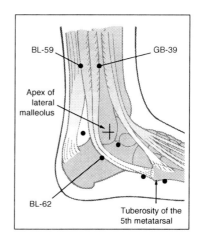

BL-59

GB-39

Apex of lateral malleolus

BL-62

Tuberosity of the 5th metatarsal

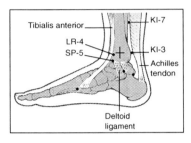

Several acupuncture points lie close to the tendons and their retinacula. GB-39 and BL-59 lie at the anterior edge and posterior edge of the peroneal muscle bellies, while BL-62 lies just posterior to the peroneal tendons within the bulk of the peroneal retinaculum. LR-4 lies just medial to the tendon of tibialis anterior between it and the anterior edge of the medial malleolus. Needling the bladder and gallbladder points in the lateral zone (see page 58) is an effective method of reducing the yang meridians. This may be balanced by reinforcing the yin meridians especially the liver and kidney. Both may be supplemented by using their source points (LR-3 and KI-3) or their tonification points (LR-8 and KI-7). Remember that by needling both meridians of an internally/externally linked pair the increased flow of qi through the channels more effectively resolves stagnation.

Massage is an effective method of supporting the removal of stagnation. Two principal methods may be used (Norris, 1998). Massage along the length of the tendons will encourage the movement of oedema within the tendon sheath. Deep frictional massage may assist with the break-up of consolidated oedema and move the tendon sheath relative to other structures allowing more normal movement. Deep frictional massage of this type is performed by placing the tendons on stretch (inversion for the peroneal tendons, for example). The practitioner places the pads of two or three fingers over the tendon and uses a to and fro movement to move the tendon over underlying tissue. The action must be movement of the tendon rather than simply rubbing the skin. The practitioner's fingers and the patient's skin must remain as one unit to avoid skin friction damage.

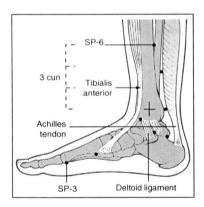

Shin pain

Shin pain occurs particularly in sport, where the term 'shin splints' is used to describe several compartment syndromes. The anterior compartment contains the tibialis anterior and the extensor muscles, the lateral compartment the peronei and the posterior compartment the flexor muscles (Fig. 8.9). Pain occurs when the muscles either hypertrophy through training or swell when inflamed. Pressure builds up as the muscle is unable to bulge, being trapped between tight skin on the outside of the body and bone and fascia on the inside. Normal resting pressure in the shin muscles is in the region of 5–10 mmHg but in shin splint conditions this pressure may raise to as much as 30–35 mmHg, reducing blood flow through the muscle. Stagnation occurs preventing waste products from escaping and nutrients from entering the muscle. The net result is pain initially with muscle degradation in severe cases.

The aim of acupuncture treatment is to activate the meridian channels travelling through the area and remove the stagnation and obstruction. As the stagnation is fluid in nature the spleen channel may effectively be targeted in medial (posterior) compartment syndrome where pain is localised along the edge of the tibia. This condition, also called medial tibial stress syndrome is the most common and potentially most debilitating form of shin splints. SP-9 is an important point in these cases both as a local point for the upper reaches of pain and for its ability to resolve dampness. SP-3 may be used as the source

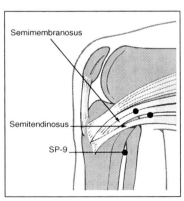

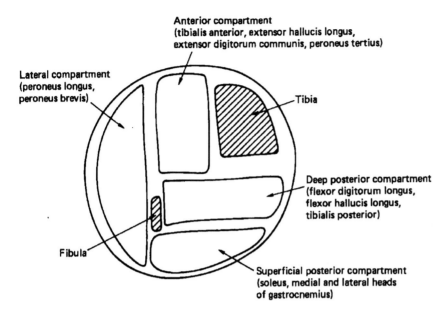

Figure 8.9. *Compartments of the lower leg*

point of the spleen meridian to encourage the flow of qi along the channel and through the painful area, and SP-6 as the meeting point of all three yin meridians of the leg. The stomach channel is the internally/externally-linked meridian and ST-36 may be used to reinforce and regulate the action of the spleen in resolving dampness. Because of the involvement of flexor hallucis longus and flexor digitorum longus, pain in this condition may travel to the toes. If this is the case either ST-41 or ST-42 may be added. ST-42 is the source point of the stomach channel but is harder to needle than ST-41. Yin channels tend towards deficiency in musculoskeletal disorders and in these conditions the presence of damp (dull aching) makes a reinforcing technique more appropriate.

For anterior shin pain the stomach meridian is chosen. This condition affects the tibialis anterior and ST-36, ST-40 and ST-41 may be usefully employed. The use of ST-36 to support the spleen in resolving dampness has been mentioned above, and the action of ST-41 to clear heat is important in this condition. ST-40 is the luo-connecting point of the stomach channel and may be used to drain excess qi. In addition ST-40 lies within the belly of tibialis anterior and may be an effective trigger point. The acupuncture treatment of posterior compartment syndrome is the same as that of a calf injury.

In parallel with acupuncture treatment training considerations in sport are also important. Excessive training of one type can be a precipitating factor and the athlete should be encouraged initially to rest totally and then to increase the variety of their training when returning to sport. Biomechanical factors in the foot, such as excessive pronation, can be important and podiatric assessment and management may be required. Muscle imbalance should also be addressed. In many cases of anterior compartment syndrome, for example, the endurance capacity of the tibialis anterior may need to be increased using repeated dorsiflexion actions to prepare the muscle for the resumption of sport. The patient should be taught self-massage to assist in the resolution of

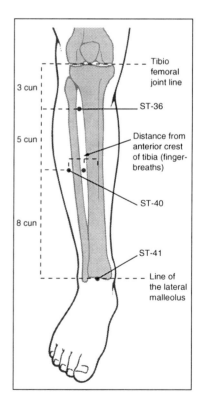

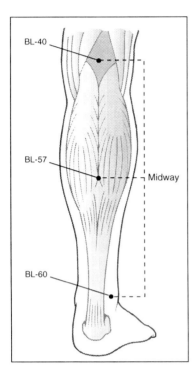

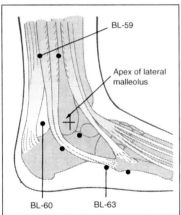

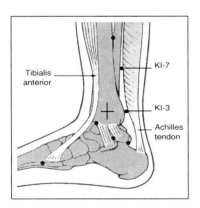

stagnation between treatment sessions. Stretching to the affected muscles is also of value.

Calf

Calf pain may occur either as a result of pain referral from the lumbar spine or through trauma to the gastrocnemius (tennis leg) or soleus. Compartment syndrome may also occur to the deep flexors (flexor digitorum longus, flexor hallucis longus and tibialis posterior). Circulatory conditions such as claudication should also be considered.

The major point for calf pain is BL-57 located in the depression formed between the two bellies of gastrocnemius. This may be supplemented by BL-40 proximally and BL-60 distally. Where the extraordinary vessels are to be brought into play BL-62 may be chosen instead and combined with SI-3 on the opposite hand. This will have the effect of opening the governing vessel and the yang motility vessel (yang qiao mai) and this is an effective combination for chronic calf pain referred from the back or leg (Seem, 1993).

Stagnation within the calf (as opposed to referred pain) may be helped by general massage and stretching to the area. Stretching into dorsiflexion with the knee straight targets the gastrocnemius, while keeping the knee bent takes the stress from the gastrocnemius and throws it onto the soleus. Placing the toes on a folded towel to force them into extension increases the stretch on the toe flexor muscles.

Achilles

The Achilles is the largest tendon in the body at some 15 cm long and about 2 cm thick. It runs from the musculotendinous junction of the calf muscles (gastrocnemius and soleus), the soleus inserting lower down on the deep surface of the tendon. The tendon gets more rounded as it descends, spreading out to insert into the posterior aspect of the calcaneum. A bursa (retrocalcaneal bursa) lies between the Achilles and the calcaneum and also (subcutaneous calcaneal bursa) between the Achilles and the skin. The Achilles is surrounded by a membranous covering called the paratenon and has lubricated membranes which lie medial and lateral to it. Fatty connective tissue lies beneath it. All of these structures act to reduce friction.

When the lubricating system breaks down and friction increases, tendonitis may result. The onset is gradual and the Achilles appears thickened compared to the tendon on the unaffected side of the body. Adhesions often develop between the Achilles and surrounding tissues and scarring can occur within the paratenon and the Achilles itself. Focal degeneration is a common occurrence in the over 30 age group and partial and complete tendon rupture in the over 40s. Rupture is more common in the less active where the Achilles has a tendency to become less pliable.

Rest is a vital component of treatment as overuse is a primary cause. Several acupuncture points are of use for treatment of the Achilles as the bladder meridian lies on the lateral aspect of the Achilles and the kidney on the medial. Both meridians are within the dorsal cutaneous

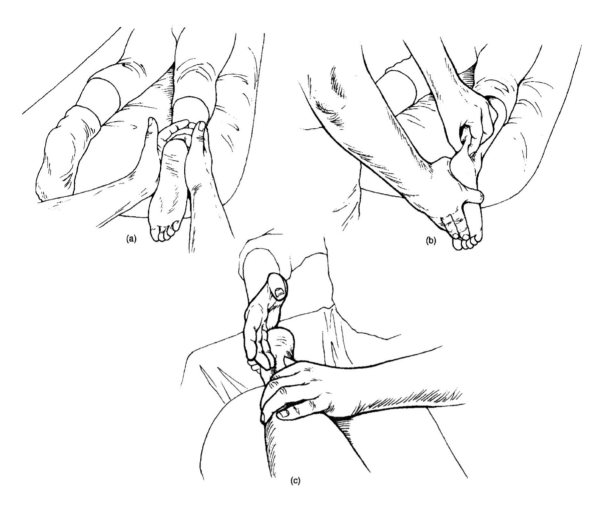

zone. Where the calf is affected together with the Achilles, the bladder meridian is chosen and BL-57 and BL-60 may be used. Where tenderness is located laterally but only on the Achilles, BL-60 may be combined with BL-59. Medial Achilles pain sees the use of KI-3 and KI-7 or KI-3 and KI-9 if the pain stretches up into the calf. In all cases, KI-3 and BL-60 may be joined by through needling, remembering that as both points lie 0.5–1.0 cun below the surface the needle need only reach to this depth below the skin on the opposite side to the insertion.

Local massage is of great benefit to resolve stagnation. General finger kneading techniques may be used along the side of the Achilles. The patient lies prone and the foot is plantarflexed over a folded towel. Pressure is applied, using one finger supported by the other, to the sides of the tendon where swelling tends to congregate. Deep transverse friction techniques may also be used. The junction of the Achilles and calcaneum (teno-osseus junction) may be treated using the sides of the flexed forefingers. The hands are pulled distally to tighten them onto the teno-osseous junction and the friction is imparted using a to and fro action of the elbows (Fig. 8.10a). The tendon itself and the junction between the tendon and the muscle (musculotendinous junction) may

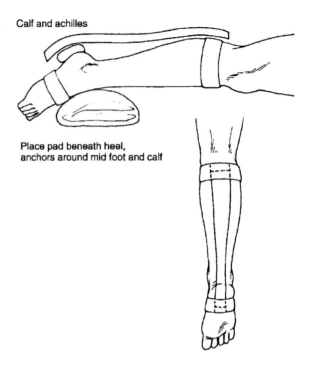

Calf and achilles

Place pad beneath heel,
anchors around mid foot and calf

Figure 8.11 *Taping the Achilles. Place elastic anchors around the mid-foot and calf, and a felt heel raise below the heel. Tape with the patient prone and the foot plantarflexed. Three reins run between the foot and calf to maintain the plantarflexed position*

be treated using a light pinch grip to hold the tendon between the forefinger and thumb (Fig. 8.10b). The patient lies prone with their foot over the end of the treatment couch and the practitioner passively dorsiflexes the foot to place the Achilles on stretch. The action is to move the hand perpendicularly to the tendon. Ensure that the skin and fingers move as a single unit rather than simply rubbing the skin. The tendon sheath and under surface of the tendon is targeted by plantarflexing the foot and moving the tendon to the side with one hand while placing the length of the fingers alongside the tendon. By pronating and supinating the practitioner's forearm a scooping action is used to friction the tendon sides (Fig. 8.10c).

Taping may be used to take the stretch off the Achilles during the irritable phase of the injury. The ankle is taped into plantarflexion with the heel on a raise (Fig. 8.11). Elastic anchor tapes are placed around the mid-foot and the top of the calf taking care not to completely encircle the limb and compromise the circulation. A heel pad is placed beneath the calcaneum (orthopaedic felt or non-compressible rubber) and three strips of taping run between the foot and calf to maintain the plantarflexed position.

Exercise plays an important part in treatment as pain subsides. The Achilles is stretched using a dorsiflexion motion with the knee bent. Typically the patient places their foot on a stool, and keeping the foot flat, presses the knee forwards to force the foot into passive dorsiflexion. Angling the knee inwards and then outwards alters the stress on the Achilles throwing the stretch on to different areas of the tendon. Following pain the calf muscle will waste and redevelopment of the calf musculature is also vital. Heel raising actions (resisted plantarflexion) either with the knee bent (soleus) or straight (gastro-

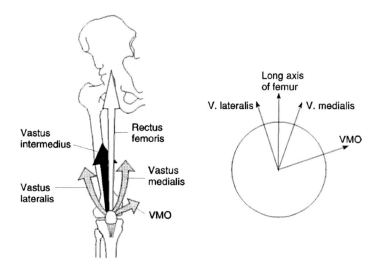

Figure 8.12. *Quadriceps pull on the patella*

cnemius) are used initially with partial weight bearing and eventually full weight bearing with or without additional resistance. In sports especially it is important to add rapid actions to develop muscle reaction speed, once normal strength has been restored. This is because the Achilles and calf combined produces force through elastic recoil as well as by active muscle contraction during rapid 'springy' movements such as jogging and jumping.

Knee

Anterior knee pain

The patella is the largest sesamoid bone in the body and as such a source of considerable discomfort for specific populations. In the adolescent anterior knee pain is common, while in middle age patella femoral arthritis is more usually seen, but the treatment approach to both conditions is broadly similar. The coordinated pull of the tissues around the patella should ensure that its path along the patellar surface of the femur is central (Fig. 8.12). An equal pull of medial and lateral structures is required. However, tight lateral structures, most notice-ably the lateral retinaculum and its attachment to the ilio-tibial band (the ilio-patellar band) often co-exist with a weakened vastus medialis muscle. The consequence is lateral deviation of the patellar path with soft tissue inflammation and bone crepitus being the end result. Alteration in either the static (at rest) or dynamic (during movement) position of the patella is therefore a contributory factor to pain, and restoration of soft tissue balance is a vital part of any management programme for patellar pain.

During the painful phase of the injury acupuncture is vital for pain relief. The Xiyan points (the lateral being ST-35) and the extra point Heding, which lies in the depression at the midpoint of the upper border of the patella, are particularly useful in this condition. The

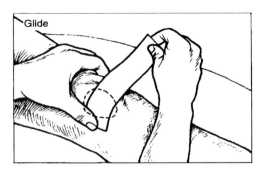

Figure 8.13. *Taping to displace the patella medially*

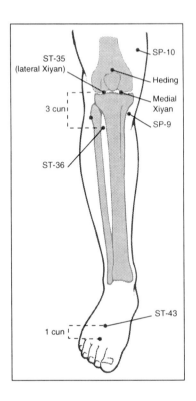

patella lies within the ventral cutaneous zone and is the yang meridian of that zone. It is supported by the spleen as the yin meridian of this zone and SP-10 in the centre of the VMO (vastus medialis obliqus) is an important point as this muscle is often inhibited and/or wasted in anterior knee pain. ST-36 may be added as a command point and ST-42 (source point) or ST-43 (easier to needle) as distal points. Where pain is mostly located over the medial aspect of the knee, SP-9 may be used in addition to SP-10 and SP-3 (source point) used as a distal point to support the yin meridian.

As pain begins to subside, the tight lateral structures must be stretched and the medial musculature restored, in an attempt to realign patella position. The practitioner may passively move the patella medially to stretch the tightened lateral structures and taping may be used to pull the patellar medially and maintain the effect between treatment sessions. With the patient supine and relaxed a piece of non-elastic tape is placed over the top of the patella and drawn tight medially (Fig. 8.13). This will also have the effect of reminding the patient of the correct patellar alignment (biofeedback) during exercise.

Optimal lower limb alignment is the key to restoration of balanced muscle function around the patella. Often patients with this condition have a combination of increased pronation of the foot ('flat foot'), medial rotation of the tibia, and adduction of the femur. This is accentuated when descending slopes and stairs in particular and this is an important factor which encourages the lateral patellar drift. To help correct the malalignment the opposite body positions are chosen. The patient stands on one leg and performs a 'mini dip' exercise. The body weight is taken onto the outside of the foot (supination) and the knee drawn laterally to lie over the centre of the foot (lateral rotation of the tibia). The action is to 'stand tall', lengthening the spine, and while maintaining this lengthened position to dip the leg and bend the knee by 20°. The knee must remain directly over the centre of the foot and not be allowed to drift medially.

Patellar tendon

Several less common sports injuries are seen around the patella. Jumper's knee is a generic term given to patellar pain. However, there are a number of injuries which may be present. Patellar tendonitis is inflammation of the patellar tendon itself. There may also be isolated damage to the attachment of the tendon to the lower pole of the patella

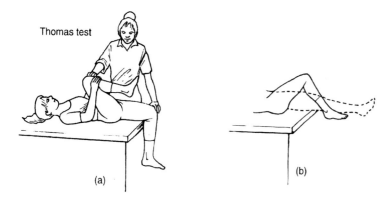

Thomas test

(a) (b)

Figure 8.14. *Thomas test. (a) Normal. (b) Tight rectus femoris—hip flexed, but femur drops down as leg is straightened*

(teno-osseous junction). The insertion itself may be inflamed and in some cases calcification may be present. Palpation of the lower pole of the patella is facilitated by extending the knee and relaxing the quadriceps. If the practitioner presses with the flat of their hand onto the top of the patella, the lower pole is brought upwards and the palpating finger is now able to touch under the bottom edge of the lower pole. In the adolescent the lower pole of the patella may separate from, or fail to properly join to, the rest of the patella; a condition called Sinding–Larsen–Johansson disease. At the other end of the patellar tendon, the insertion onto the tibia may be affected. Again this is seen in adolescents when it is called Osgood-Schlatter's syndrome. The patella tendon insertion onto the tibial tubercle is disrupted causing the tubercle to partially separate from the tibial shaft.

Two acupuncture approaches may be used. The Xiyan points lie on either side of the patellar tendon within the patellar fat pads. Needling them in combination with ST-36 and ST-34 can be of use. Periosteal needling may be used to the tibial tubercle and to the lower pole of the patella with reasonable results.

Whichever procedure is used, stretching is an essential part of the patient's home care. Lying supine and pulling the knee to the chest (maximum knee flexion) will stretch the tendon, while targeting the rectus femoris muscle is also important if this muscle is found to be tight. To assess tightness in the anterior thigh the Thomas test is used (Fig. 8.14). The subject should move to the end of the examination couch so that the backs of the knees clear the couch end. Both knees are bent and the feet placed on the couch. The opposite knee to the painful patella is pulled into the chest and held. The painful leg is then straightened. If the anterior thigh muscles are of normal length the painful leg will rest down on the couch with the femur on the couch and the tibia vertical (Fig. 8.14a). If the thigh muscles are tight the thigh is held above the surface of the couch (Fig. 8.14b). Bending and straightening the knee further localises the tightness. This exercise may then be used to stretch the muscle with the patient holding the uninjured knee to the chest for 30–60 seconds and allowing the injured leg to gradually descend to the couch. An additional exercise is to stand close to a wall and to bend the knee and pull the femur backwards into extension (Fig. 8.15). With this exercise care must be taken to keep the back straight. Hollowing the back takes the stress off the leg and throws it onto the lumbar spine instead.

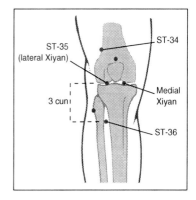

ST-35 (lateral Xiyan)

ST-34

Medial Xiyan

3 cun

ST-36

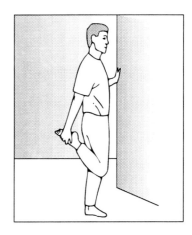

Figure 8.15. *Anterior thigh stretch*

Knee arthritis

Knee arthritis tends to give pain either anteriorly in which case the patella femoral joint is implicated (see above) or medially over the course of the yin meridians of the leg (within the ventral cutaneous zone). Deficiency of the kidney, liver and spleen could occur, with the kidney being the most likely, as the kidney organ dominates the bones. Knee pain due to kidney deficiency must be differentiated from that due to bi syndrome. With that due to kidney deficiency the pain is usually bilateral and the knee feels cold. It is rarely swollen and not necessarily affected by the weather. If due to bi syndrome there may be swelling due to the invasion of pathogenic cold and damp and the pain often occurs suddenly (although an underlying kidney deficiency may already exist) and is generally made worse by damp cold wintry weather.

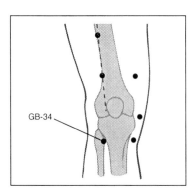

The kidney and spleen channels are targeted in treatment, and both KI-3 (source point) and KI-7 (tonification point and river point) may be used. GB-34 (influential point for sinews) is used to ease pain and stiffness in the joint in general, and if the pain is located *laterally* other gallbladder points GB-40 (source point) may be added. For pain positioned *anteriorly* stomach points may be chosen. River points are said to affect joints, being the points where an external pathogen travelling up the meridians may move deeper and enter the joints and tissues (see page 65), and so both ST-41 and SP-5 (both river points) may be used. ST-41 for anterior pain and SP-5 for *medial* pain, especially that involving dampness. Where the knee is heavily swollen, SP-9 may also be added.

Where the knee is one of several joints affected by the arthritis, more general treatment may be selected and BL-23 (back shu point of the kidney) and BL-11 (influential point of bones) may be added.

Periosteal acupuncture may be used in cases of pain over the medial aspect of the knee and especially the medial joint line. The medial aspect of the tibia, anterior to SP-9 (the pes anserine region) may be targeted, and the medial joint line itself. Any tender areas are needled, and sensation may radiate downwards along the medial aspect of the shin, and into the knee joint itself. A 'peppering' or 'pecking' technique is used where the needle is inserted until bone contact is made. The needle is withdrawn slightly from the bone (but not from the skin) and inserted at a different angle until bone is again struck. The procedure may be repeated several times.

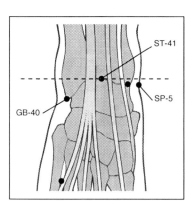

Joint and soft tissue mobilisation procedures, together with exercise, provide additional tools which the practitioner must have to effectively treat knee arthritis. Soft tissue techniques include massage along the joint line and frictional massage to the coronary ligament, the attachment of the meniscus to the tibial plateaux. This procedure is performed with the knee flexed to 90° and the tibia externally rotated. This position brings the edge of the tibial plateaux forwards enabling the palpating finger to touch the coronary ligament. The action is a horizontal movement along the edge of the joint line. Joint mobilisation in cases of knee arthritis attempts to restore the accessory movement or 'joint play' to the joint. These are movements which the patient cannot perform with his/her own joint but which can be performed on the joint passively. They are vital for pain-free function of any joint. A number of techniques are available but the 'capsular stretch' is of particular benefit during chronic episodes of arthritis. For this procedure the patient's knee is flexed and the practitioner places his forearm in the crook of the knee to provide a fulcrum for the knee to flex around. The mobilisation is a gentle rhythmical oscillation gradually increasing the range of motion to flexion.

Exercise for the knee following an acute episode of pain from arthritis focuses on the quadriceps musculature which tends to waste through disuse and may also suffer pain inhibition. It should be emphasised however that all of the knee muscles should be re-strengthened eventually, during the later stages of rehabilitation, and it is a gross error to strengthen the quadriceps alone. Initially exercise begins non weight bearing (foot off the ground). Simply sitting on a bench or table and straightening (extending) the knee is sufficient to begin with. The patient should be encouraged to lock the knee out completely and to hold this position for 3–5 seconds. As this becomes easier some resistance should be used to challenge (overload) the muscles. This may be a heavy folded towel placed over the ankle or a lightweight bag of the type available in most sports shops. The patient should aim to perform 10–12 repetitions holding the leg straight for 3–5 seconds each time. The patient should then progress to partial weight-bearing exercises (foot on the floor, taking some bodyweight through the arms or other leg) and eventually full weight bearing (the injured limb taking all of the bodyweight). Slow actions are progressed gradually to faster movements such as hopping and jumping, for example. For details of knee rehabilitation see Norris (1998).

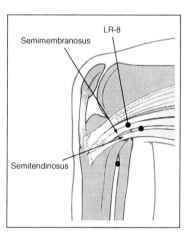

Knee ligament injuries

Several knee ligaments may be injured commonly but the medial collateral ligament (MCL) on the inside of the knee joint is the most likely to give problems in everyday clinical practice. The MCL is a broad flat band about 8 cm long. It travels forwards and downwards from the medial epicondyle of the femur to the medial condyle and shaft of the tibia. The ligament has both deep and superficial fibres, the deep fibres attaching to the medial meniscus (inner knee 'cartilage').

The point LR-8 lies on the posterior edge of the MCL at the level of the joint line. This point is often painful to palpation and may be needled together with ahshi points along the length of the MCL. Where LR-8 is selected it may be combined with LR-3 as a distal point. GB-34 may also be chosen as the influential point of sinews and also because the liver and gallbladder channels are internally/externally related.

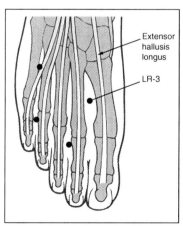

Local massage may be used to supplement acupuncture treatment, and altering the angle of knee flexion can be used to differentiate between the deep and superficial portions of the ligament. Frictional massage may be used to assist in moving the ligament across the bone beneath, and to encourage the development of a mobile scar within the ligament as it heals. Performing the massage with the knee straight targets the superficial portion of the MCL. Using the same technique with the knee bent to 90° relaxes the superficial part of the ligament enabling the massaging finger to target the deep portion of the ligament more effectively. The action in each case is a broad sweep across the breadth of the ligament moving the practitioner's fingers and the patient's skin as one unit. The level at which the fingers are positioned is dependent on pain, with the joint line and lower insertion onto the tibia being the two most common sites.

Rehabilitation progresses as before from non weight bearing through partial weight bearing and ultimately to taking full bodyweight through the knee. The difference is that as the ligament limits valgus stresses (inward bowing) and rotation, these stresses are introduced to the knee more gradually. Standing on the injured leg and slowly twisting the body while keeping the foot on the floor will gradually challenge rotatory stability of the knee. Standing on one leg and stepping sideways (to the side and then across the front of the body) with the other knee, will challenge valgus stability. Each action should be hard enough to comfortably pull on the inside of the knee but not so severe as to cause pain.

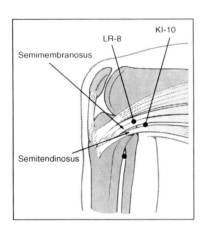

Thigh

Muscle tears to the upper leg are common in many sports. Hamstring injuries tend to occur with sprinting and quadriceps tears through kicking actions. The adductors may be injured with any side-stepping action which causes a sudden overstretch. The hamstrings, rectus femoris, and the gracilis (an accessory adductor) are the three muscles from the group which are injured most readily through trauma. They are biarticular muscles (they act over two joints), in this case the knee and the hip. The coordinated action of a biarticular muscle is complex (See Norris, 1998, pp. 17 and 155–159). When this coordination breaks down through fatigue or training imbalances, injury may result. Again, acupuncture goes hand in hand with other forms of physical medicine treatment.

Injury to the hamstrings may occur in one of three sites, to the tendons at the knee, the origin at the ischial tuberosity or within the main muscle belly. The points LR-8 and KI-10 both lie close to the semitendinosus and semimembranosus tendons at the knee and may be used as local points. BL-39 lies medial to the tendon of the biceps femoris at the level of the popliteal crease and again may be chosen as a local point. Mid and upper belly tears may be targeted by needling BL-37 and BL-36. For a tear affecting the ishial tuberosity BL-36 may be used and the needle angled superiorly towards the ischial tuberosity. These points may be supplemented with BL-40 and BL-60 as distal points.

A differential diagnosis must be made for pain in the posterior thigh. If the pain is neural in origin, the slump test will usually be positive. For this test the patient sits on the couch end, flexes their neck (chin to chest) and 'slumps' or flexes the spine as though trying to place their nose onto their umbilicus. This action is combined with straightening the leg and dorsiflexing the ankle. If this reproduces posterior leg pain the head is lifted (extended) from its flexed position to neutral to see what effect this has on the pain. If the thigh pain is reduced, the test is positive and the pain is of neural origin. Clearly straightening the head releases some tension on the neural tissues but does not alter the position of either the pelvis or the knee, both bones to which the

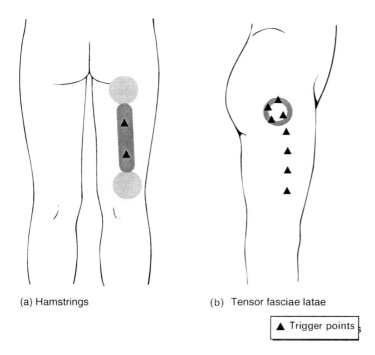

(a) Hamstrings   (b) Tensor fasciae latae

▲ Trigger points

Figure 8.16. *Patterns of pain referral from upper leg muscle trigger points. (**a**) Hamstrings. (**b**) Tensor fasciae latae. (Reproduced with permission from Baldrey, 1998)*

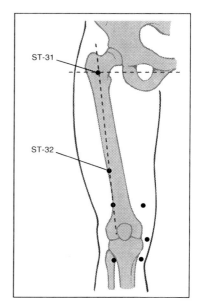

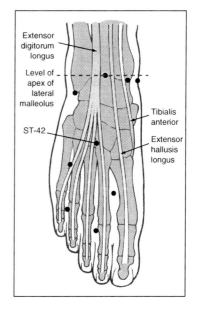

hamstrings attach. If the test is negative, (thigh pain remains as the head is raised), resisted knee flexion confirms the hamstring muscle involvement. Where hamstring pain exists, even though it is made worse through muscle contraction, palpation or straight leg raising, these tests do not by themselves prove muscle damage. Active trigger points in the hamstrings (Fig. 8.16a) may refer pain down towards the knee or up towards the buttock. Palpation is used to differentiate trauma from trigger points. A positive jump sign (see page 122) confirms the trigger point and local needling should readily diminish the pain. Muscle trauma and internal scarring (stagnation in TCM terms) will take far longer to clear, and may be helped with distal points as well as massage.

Periosteal needling may be used directly over the ischial tuberosity but the starting position is modified. Traditionally upper posterior thigh points are needled with the patient prone, but periosteal treatment is better carried out with the patient in side lying with the affected leg on top and drawn up. This stretches the soft tissue and reduces the distance from the needle to the bone. Once inserted and bone contact is made, the needle is partially withdrawn and re-inserted to give a 'peppering' effect over the whole ischial origin of the hamstrings.

Injury to the rectus femoris may be localised to the mid belly over the anterior thigh or to the muscle origins at the anterior inferior iliac spine or above the acetabulum. For mid and upper belly tears blood stagnation may be cleared by activating the stomach channel using ST-31 and ST-32 locally and ST-42 distally. A periosteal technique aimed at the anterior superior iliac spine may be used for the upper insertion of the rectus and for the sartorius, and this local point may refer pain along the whole of the upper part of the muscle. The needle may be

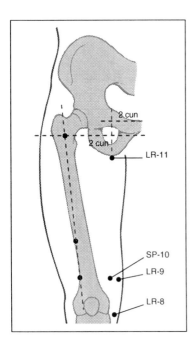

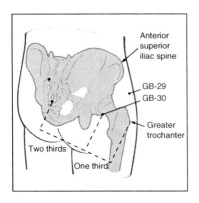

inserted either from above perpendicular to the skin, or in lean subjects from a medial approach parallel to the skin.

Injury to the adductor muscles will give pain on resisted adduction and pain to adductor stretching. Pain is made worse for the gracilis (the only adductor to pass below the knee) if abduction is carried out with the knee straight rather than bent. Both the liver and kidney meridians are related to the adductors. The kidney channel runs from KI-10 at the medial side of the popliteal fossa along the postero-medial aspect of the inner thigh to the tip of the coccyx. The liver channel runs from LR-8 anterior to the semitendinosis to the pubic region. Both the kidney and liver sinew channels are situated on the adductor aspect of the inner thigh with the kidney lying slightly posterior to the liver. Both sinew channels bind over the medial aspect of the knee and at the pubic region. Local treatment targets ahshi points in the upper adductor region and LR-11 lies on the anterior border of adductor longus. This point lies 2 cun lateral to the midline, and 2 cun below the upper surface of the pubic symphasis. It may be combined with LR-9 and this combination is also suitable for sartorius involvement as the point lies 2 cun above the upper border of the patella in the depression between vastus medialis and sartorius.

Where pain is located directly over the pubic ramus calcification (osteitis pubis) must be eliminated in chronic conditions. CV-2 lies over the superior border of the symphasis pubis and this whole area may be palpated for tender periosteal points. Disruption of the symphasis through trauma must also be eliminated as a possible cause of pain. In each case the acupuncture treatment may be similar but any manual therapy techniques used will differ.

A variety of physical therapy techniques are available to the practitioner treating groin injury including soft tissue manipulation, pelvic adjustment procedures, and muscle energy techniques. Stretching exercises should form part of the treatment and Fig. 8.17 shows examples of stretches for the adductors, rectus femoris and hamstrings. For mid belly muscle tears re-strengthening the muscle is also important. Strength exercises, as well as reversing any muscle wasting, will allow the muscle to broaden and disrupt any consolidated oedema and adhesive scarring between the individual muscle fibres.

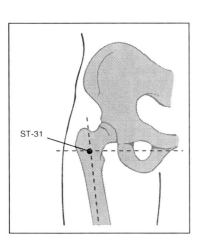

Hip

The hip joint responds well to acupuncture treatment with the pain from mild to moderately severe coxa femoral arthritis being cleared completely in many cases. The main meridians affected are the gallbladder whose sinew channel extends from the lateral aspect of the hip across the buttock to the sacrum, the spleen (important where medial pain is present) whose sinew channel binds over the anterior aspect of the hip, and the stomach whose regular meridian ascends to ST-31 directly over the neck of the femur. Points on the gallbladder channel include GB-30 as the main posterior local point with GB-29 as the lateral point. These may be supplemented by GB-31 if the pain extends along the lateral aspect of the leg and GB-40 as the source point of the gallbladder channel. GB-34 (influential point of sinews)

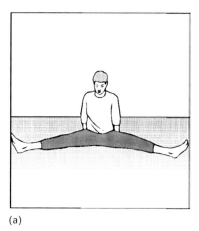
(a)

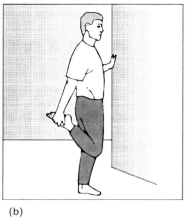
(b)

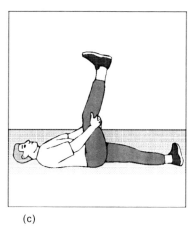
(c)

may be used as a distal point where soft tissue pain is the overpowering feature. GB-39 (influential point for marrow) may be used instead to target the joint where chronic bisyndrome is present and gross muscle weakness is present. ST-31 is a useful anterior point. Its Chinese name (Biguan) means 'thigh gate' and this point may be seen as the equivalent point to LI-15 in the upper limb. Both points are important to regulate blood and qi in the whole limb (Deadman et al., 1998).

A number of extra points have been said to exist, one on the lateral aspect of the femur just below the greater trochanter (Low, 1987) and three points superior, anterior and posterior to the greater trochanter (Ellis et al., 1994). Any local points may be needled if painful, and several trigger points have been identified in and around the trochanter and along the upper portion of the tensor fascia lata and ilio-tibial band (Baldrey, 1998). The use of moxibustion and warm needling is particularly helpful in cases of painful and chronic bisyndrome where the pain is worse in cold damp weather.

Joint mobilisation procedures are an important parallel to acupuncture treatment of the hip. Longitudinal mobilisation and general hip traction is especially beneficial. For this procedure the patient lies supine and the hip is placed into its open pack position (the position where the deep soft tissues are relaxed) with the hip slightly flexed, abducted and externally rotated. The practitioner grasps the patient's ankle or lower shin (pad the area with a folded towel) and leans back to provide traction. The movement must be gradual without any snapping action to begin or recoil to finish. More specific mobilisation procedures may be used by grasping the thigh and directing the force longitudinally or laterally. Capsular stretching is also of benefit. When very inflamed the hip tends to be held slightly flexed, tightening the anterior capsule of the joint. Initially, simply lying on the front on a firm surface (towel on the floor rather than on a bed) will stretch the anterior joint. An additional stretch may be gained by lying on the back with the thigh over the bed end. The unaffected knee is drawn up towards the chest (tilting the pelvis backwards and flattening the lumbar spine) and the weight of the affected leg gradually draws it downwards towards the horizontal.

Figure 8.17. *Stretching the upper leg muscles. (a) Sit in a stride position with the arms behind to stretch the adductors. Push on the floor with the hands to straighten the spine and keep it straight throughout the movement. (b) Stand facing the wall and grip the ankle. Bend the knee and pull the thigh backwards (hip extension) without arching the spine. (c) Lie on the floor and grip behind one knee. Use the thigh muscles (quadriceps) to straighten the legs and stretch the hamstrings*

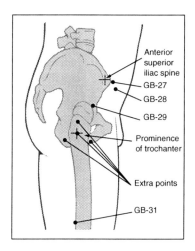

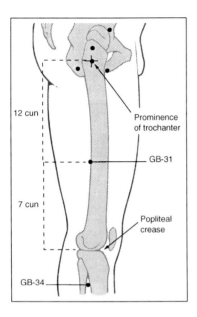

12 cun

Prominence
of trochanter

GB-31

7 cun

Popliteal
crease

GB-34

ITB friction syndrome

Friction syndromes of the ilio-tibial band (ITB) are common in endurance sports. They can occur at the upper end of the ITB over the greater trochanter or at the lower end over the femoral epicondyle (see page 155). The fault usually lies with tightness in the ITB and over-activity in the tensor fascia latae muscle which may develop several trigger points (Fig. 8.16b). In standing the ITB lies posterior to the hip joint axis and anterior to the knee joint axis. As the knee flexes past 30° the ITB passes posterior to the knee axis and in so doing glides over the lateral epicondyle of the femur. With flexion of the hip the greater trochanter moves in front of the ITB and with extension it moves back beneath it. If tight, the ITB will develop friction as it passes over these two points. GB-33 may be used as a local point for ITB friction syndrome around the knee and extra points over the greater trochanter (see above) for ITB friction syndrome over the hip. GB-31 may be used where pain and tightness occur in the ITB itself. Distal points are selected from the gallbladder meridian, typically GB-34 and GB-40.

Stretching of the ITB should also be used in parallel with acupuncture treatment. Stretching is achieved by holding the pelvis firm (avoiding any sideways tipping) and adducting the leg. This may be conducted in standing or lying.

Piriformis syndrome

The piriformis muscle attaches from the front of the sacrum, the inner surface of the pelvis and the sacrotuberous ligament and travels through the greater sciatic notch to the medial aspect of the greater trochanter. It therefore touches the sciatic nerve and in some individuals is divided into two so that the nerve actually passes through it. If the piriformis tightens and develops trigger points it can affect conduction in the sciatic nerve explaining the length of pain referral that it can create (Fig. 8.18). The muscle can be palpated along a line from the greater trochanter to the 2nd, 3rd, and 4th sacral segments and a number of trigger points may be found in this region. The points BL-54, BL-28 and GB-30 lie in close proximity to the muscle, but clinically it is often more effective to select the tender local points, (especially if they reproduce the patient's symptoms), rather than the traditional points.

Following treatment the muscle may be stretched using a combination of hip flexion, abduction and internal rotation. The stretch should be maintained for 30–60 seconds.

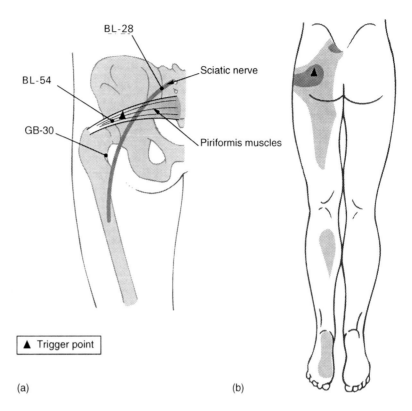

BL-28

BL-54

GB-30

Sciatic nerve

Piriformis muscles

▲ Trigger point

Figure 8.18. *Piriformis pain. (a) Muscle position in relation to acupuncture points. (b) Pattern of pain referral*

(a)

(b)

9

Back and trunk treatment protocols

Lower back

Low back pain (LBP) is the most common complaint that brings patients into the clinic. It is said that four out of five individuals will suffer from LBP at some time in their lives and this staggering number presents the practitioner with a tremendous clinical challenge. For effective management of these conditions it is *essential* that acupuncture be combined with other forms of physical therapy including manual therapy of some type and exercise therapy. The combination of these three can successfully manage LBP in full, leaving the patient fully functional rather than simply pain free.

The true pathology which gives rise to LBP has never been completely described, and a variety of anatomical structures have been implicated as sources of pain. The lumbar disc is often the primary culprit in terms of medical diagnosis. However, lumbar disc lesions have been found in as many as 50 per cent of normal individuals (Bowden et al., 1990), so the presence of the lesion itself cannot be the only feature to determine pain. Although radiographic changes in the lumbar spine are often used to determine treatment from a medical perspective, these changes are also highly unreliable. It has been claimed that as many individuals without pain show evidence of disc degeneration on X-ray as those with pain (Nachemson, 1992). The practitioner is therefore left with pain description (subjective) and functional measures/tests (objective) as perhaps the most reliable indicators of the effect of pathology and the outcome of treatment.

Facet joints

The facet (zygopophyseal) joints are synovial joints formed between the articular processes of two neighbouring vertebrae (Fig. 9.1). They have a loose capsule strengthened by the ligamentum flavum and reinforced by the multifidus muscle. Above and below each joint are small pockets

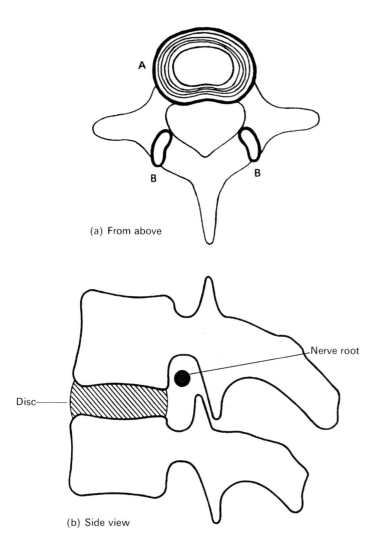

(a) From above

Disc

Nerve root

(b) Side view

Figure 9.1. *Lumbar vertebra.* **(a)** *The mobile intervertebral joint, seen from above, is composed of the intervertebral disc (A) in front and the two zygopophyseal joints (B) behind.* **(b)** *The intervertebral foramen with its nerve root is bounded in front by the intervertebral disc and vertebral bodies, above and below by the pedicles, and behind by the zygopophyseal joint. (Reproduced with permission from Corrigan and Maitland, 1998)*

acting as reservoirs for fat droplets which are moved in and out of the joint as it opens and closes. Small tissue pads also exist to further protect the joint cartilage as the facet joint moves. As the spine moves the facet joints open and close, and are subjected to both compression (squeezing) and shear (gliding) forces which may disrupt any of the joint structures. With age the joints can develop arthritis, making them less able to cope with the stresses imposed upon them.

Each facet joint of the lumbar spine may be palpated through the thick spinal muscles about 1 cm lateral and slightly below the spinous process. Extension movements impact (close) the joint surfaces while flexion tractions (opens) the joints. With the patient lying prone, if the lumbar lordosis (curve) is excessive the spine is extended, tending to compress the facets and increase pain where facet pathology is present. Placing a pillow or roll under the stomach will flatten the lordosis, flexing the lumbar spine and opening the facets. In the thoracic spine the facet joints are close to the articulations of the ribs, making differentiation by palpation extremely difficult.

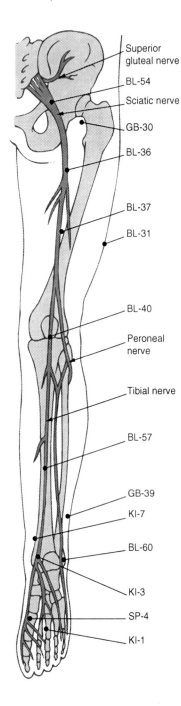

Superior gluteal nerve

BL-54

Sciatic nerve

GB-30

BL-36

BL-37

BL-31

BL-40

Peroneal nerve

Tibial nerve

BL-57

GB-39

KI-7

BL-60

KI-3

SP-4

KI-1

Figure 9.2. *Course of the sciatic nerve in relation to acupuncture points*

Lumbar discs

There are 24 spinal discs lying between successive vertebrae, those of the lumbar spine being thicker than those higher up. The lumbar discs may be as much as 10 mm thick (Fig. 9.1). The disc consists of a spongy central region (nucleus palposis) surrounded by about 20 concentric outer rings (annulus fibrosis). The discs provide shock absorption to the spine with both compression and movement. A 100 kg load on the spine has been shown to compress the lumbar discs by 1.4 mm and expand them sideways by 0.75 mm (Hirsch and Nachemson, 1954). With continuous loading water is slowly squeezed out of the disc making the patient 'shrink'. For example, in sport the loads involved in training may have a noticeable effect on the lumbar spine. Weight training, for example, has been shown to lead to height losses of 5.4 mm and a 6 km run reduced height by 3.25 mm (Leatt et al., 1986). Repeated bending (flexion) movements on the lumbar spine have been claimed to have a pumping action on the lumbar disc. The nucleus palposis of the disc is said to gradually move backwards, stretching the posterior wall of the disc and causing it to bulge (McKenzie, 1981).

The discal movements described above are important for pathology. The spinal cord runs the length of the spine from the brain to the lumbar region. At each spinal level nerves emerge at 'T junctions' forming nerve roots (Fig 9.1). The nerve root lies close to the back of the disc and any compression force which causes the disc to bulge has the potential of pressing the disc onto the nerve root causing pain. This pain may be experienced locally in the lumbar spine, but also wherever the nerve runs. In the case of the sciatic nerve this is down the back of the leg to the foot, and in the case of the femoral nerve the anterior thigh. Several acupuncture points in the bladder, gallbladder and kidney meridians lie in close proximity to the sciatic nerve and its branches and may be used effectively to treat referred lumbar pain of this type (Fig. 9.2).

TCM models of low back pain

The bladder and kidney channels are the most important with reference to LBP. The inner and outer bladder channels run the length of the spine and the kidney channel goes deeper into the body at the perineum and flows along the spine and into the kidney organ. The kidney divergent channel joins the Girdle vessel (extra meridian) at the point BL-23, and the penetrating vessel (extra meridian) sends a branch to the spine at this point (Maciocia, 1994). In addition, BL-23 is the back shu point of the kidney making this point especially important in the treatment of LBP. The governing vessel runs the length of the spine centrally and points such as GV-4 (gate of life) may be used to nourish the kidneys especially in cases of chronic LBP in the elderly. It should be noted that both of these points are level with L2 (second lumbar vertebra), GV-4 centrally and BL-23 1.5 cun laterally.

The three most common presentations of LBP are kidney deficiency (chronic), stagnation of qi and blood (soft tissue injury) and retention of cold and damp (bi syndrome). Kidney deficiency gives chronic LBP

Table 9.1. TCM models of low back pain.

Kidney deficiency	Stagnation (blood and qi)	Pathogen (cold and damp)
Chronic condition typical in the elderly.	Well localised area, 'sprain'.	Worse in cold damp weather, better when sunny and warm.
May underly other (acute) conditions.	Sharp stabbing pains with muscle spasm.	System weak (kidney deficiency) allowing pathogenic invasion.
Dull ache, not well localised.	Better with movement as stagnation is 'worked loose'. Worse through the day.	Better in the morning, and with rest. Pain worse with pressure (palpation).
Pain eased by pressure (palpation).		Trigger points and many ahshi points.

which is dull and aching in nature. It is better with rest and worse with overexertion. There may be a deficiency of kidney yang (warming) and so the area may feel cold to the touch. Kidney deficiency itself leaves the back open to pathogenic attack and often underlies other more acute conditions. Supporting the kidney (yin channel) when using bladder points (yang channel) to treat acute pain is therefore important.

Differentiation is made by questioning and observation (Table 9.1). The patient with kidney deficiency often has a pale complexion and complains of dull aching rather than stabbing pain (which would indicate stagnation). The pain of kidney deficiency improves with rest (allowing energy to build up) while that of stagnation requires gentle exercise to encourage the flow of qi and blood. Deficiency pain is generally better in the morning and gets worse through the day as energy is used up.

Stagnation pain is the opposite, lack of movement overnight leads to increased stagnation and so the pain is worse in the morning and is gradually 'worked loose' through the day. Pain which is worse in cold damp weather indicates bi syndrome. In cases of kidney deficiency palpation often shows little resistance to pressure (poor muscle tone) with noticeable wasting. Spasm and stiffness indicates stagnation of blood and qi, and often the affected area is quite small, the pain being well localised (the pain is 'just there').

Invasion of a pathogen in bi syndrome usually affects the whole of the lumbar region in general, with the patient unable to accurately localise the pain (the pain is 'in that area'). Pain from deficiency requires reinforcing needling and moxibustion. In the acute phase of either pathogenic invasion or stagnation reducing needling should be used. Local bladder points should be combined with both distal bladder and kidney points.

Acupuncture treatment

Local points in the lumbar region include BL-23 (back shu points of kidney) and GV-4 (gate of life) as detailed above. Any of the Governor vessel points should be used if tender as they overly the interspinous ligament, a source of pain with prolonged flexion activities. BL-25 and BL-26 level with L4 and L5, respectively, should also be palpated and needled if painful. The extra point Shiqizhuixia is useful. This lies below

Clinical note

Palpation of the lumbar spine

The lumbar vertebrae may be located relative to the pelvic rim. A horizontal line taken across from the highest point of the iliac crests represents the *Supracristal plane*. The 4th lumbar vertebra (L4) lies level with this plane, and as the spinous processes are angled downwards the palpating finger will touch the lower border of the L3 spinous process.

The extra point Shiqizhuixia lies below the spinous process of L5. This is located by sliding the palpating finger cephalically from the sacrum along the midline. The point lies in the first hollow of the lumbar spine that the finger falls into.

The spinal cord lies between 1.25 and 1.75 cun deep depending on body build. Central points (Governor vessel) should only be inserted to 0.5–1.0 cun depth therefore. For safety always select a 1 cun needle and never insert it fully.

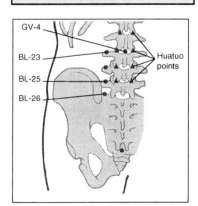

Needling the lateral side or
tip of a spinous process

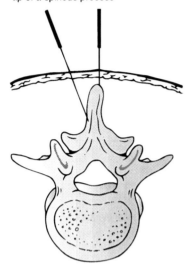

Figure 9.3. *Periosteal needling of the spinous processes*

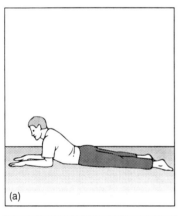

(a)

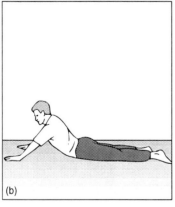

(b)

Figure 9.4. *McKenzie extension exercises for the lumbar spine*

the spinous process of L5, and the Huatuo points lateral to the depressions below the spinous process may also be used as these lie within the multifidus muscle.

Local periosteal needling may also be useful, especially where pain is well localised. Needling the spinous process either at its tip or its lateral side has been described (Mann, 1992). The needle is inserted slightly laterally to the tip of the spinous process and angled inwards aiming to strike the lateral aspect of the process at a depth of about 0.5–1.0 cun (Fig. 9.3). The radiation from periosteal needling of this type to the lower lumbar spine may travel downwards and outwards as far as the iliac crest.

Where pain travels out to the hip, select GB-30. If this pain travels laterally down the leg, GB-31 may be used and GB-34 selected as a distal point and as the influential point of sinews. Points on the sacrum may be selected for sacro-iliac pain (see below) and also for pain referred into this area. Distal points along the bladder meridian include BL-36 for pain referred only as far as the upper leg, BL-40 for referred pain to the knee and BL-60 for pain into the foot. BL-62 (confluence point) may be chosen instead to bring in the yang motility vessel and is especially useful for pain in both the lumbar region and hip. This point may be combined with SI-3 for this purpose.

There are two major approaches which may be used to augment acupuncture. The first (McKenzie approach) aims to 'squeeze the lumbar disc back into shape' after repeated flexion movements (bending or lifting). With this approach repeated flexion is seen as pushing the nucleus of the disc posteriorly towards the back wall of the disc. This causes discal bulging and impingement onto the nerve root. Repeated extension movements are therefore used in an attempt to restore balance to the disc. Patients lie on the floor in a 'press up' position and passively extend their spine by pressing with their hands. Initially they may press up onto their forearms and eventually up until the arms are straight. In each case the hips should stay on the ground and the lumbar spine is encouraged to extend (Fig. 9.4). If the patient experienced pain in the leg going down to the knee, the aim is to shrink the pain up the leg towards the hip and eventually to the spine, even if the pain gets worse (more intense). This phenomenon is called 'centralisation' and is seen as an important stage in the healing process.

The second approach is the use of joint mobilisation to reduce pain and restore movement to the lumbar spine. Side lying positions are often chosen and most patients find them more comfortable. This may be either crook side lying (both knees bent) or ½ crook side lying (top leg only bent) which places greater rotation on the spine. The practitioner stands behind the patient and gently rocks the pelvis to produce oscillatory rotation movements in the lumbar spine (Fig. 9.5a). Extension mobilisations may be performed with the patient lying prone. The practitioner uses the sides of his/her hands (pisiform bone) to press on the spinous processes or over the region of the facet joints to impart local extension or rotation to the lumbar spine (Fig 9.5b).

Exercises for the lumbar spine in addition to those described above include general mobility and strength. A variety of exercises are available and readers are referred to Norris (2000) for an in depth description of this topic. An example of a simple mobility exercise is to lie on the ground with the knees bent and slowly lower the knees to one side and the arms to the other (Fig. 9.6a). The hamstring muscles may

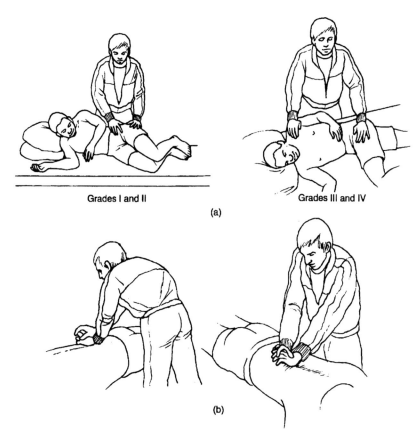

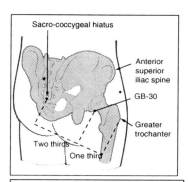

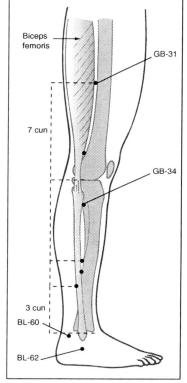

Figure 9.5. *Lumbar spine mobilisation.* **(a)** *Rotation and* **(b)** *extension*

also benefit from stretching and a suitable exercise is shown in Fig. 9.6b. This type of exercise is important because it will also place stretch on the sciatic nerve, and neural tension (tightness in nerves, usually secondary to injury) is often a limiting factor in low back conditions once the acute pain has eased.

Re-strengthening the lumbar spine following injury targets the stabilising system of this area (Norris, 1995). The deep abdominal muscles (transversus abdominis and internal oblique) contract as a type of 'deep muscle corset', to support the spine and prevent excessive motion. Exercises begin with abdominal hollowing actions, drawing the abdominal wall inwards without holding the breath. This forms the stable base upon which the limbs may move. The abdominal hollowing action is held for 10–20 seconds and then leg and arm movements are used to increase the stress imposed on the corset muscles. Examples are given in Fig. 9.7.

The sacro-iliac joint

The sacro-iliac joint (SIJ) lies between the sacrum and the sacral surfaces of the pelvis. The sacrum and two pelvic bones form a ring with the pubic joint anterior and the SIJ posterior. Disruption of the

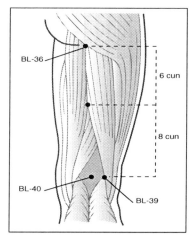

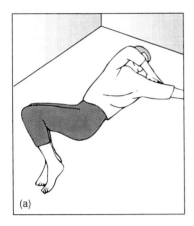

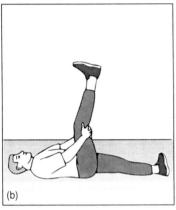

Figure 9.6. *Stretching exercises for lumbar pain.*

SIJ invariably affects the pubis and this area must be examined as part of a general musculoskeletal examination of the region. Minimal movement is available at the SIJ with greater amounts being available during non weight bearing actions. As much as 12° of pelvic rotation on the sacrum has been observed during non weight bearing flexion and 8 mm of translation during extension (Lavignolle et al., 1983). Greater movement of the SIJ is seen during childbirth, and ligamentous laxity resulting from increased Relaxin hormone concentration in the months following childbirth leave the joint less stable. Irritation of the SIJ (sacroiliitis) may give pain, as can increased (hypermobility) or decreased ('blockage' or hypomobility) movement ranges. A variety of tests may be used to examine the area (Norris, 1998) including motion tests and pelvic springing. Motion tests observe (by palpation) movement of the posterior superior iliac spine (PSIS) in leg lifting and trunk flexion movements. Asymmetry of movement of the PSIS shows a positive test. Pelvic springing (stress tests) aims to reproduce the patient's symptoms by approximating or gapping the joint. The practitioner presses on the pelvic rim or sacrum attempting to disrupt the joint. Stress testing may also be carried out using greater leverage with the ' 4 test' or FABER manoeuvre (Flexion, ABduction, External Rotation). The patient lies supine and the practitioner flexes, abducts, and externally rotates the patient's hip to place one foot above the opposite knee. Downward pressure on the knee of the bent leg stresses the SIJ on the opposite side.

The SIJ corresponds to approximately BL-27 and BL-28 and these points may be used if tender. In addition the SIJ may be needled directly (periosteal needling) to treat both local and referred pain. The joint line of the SIJ passes from a point 5 cm (2.0 cun) lateral to the 5th lumbar vertebra (L5) downwards at an angle of 25° to the posterior inferior iliac spine (PIIS). In addition the centre of the SIJ line lies 1 cm (0.5–0.8 cun) lateral to the PSIS and extends approximately 2 cm (1.0–1.5 cun) above and below this point.

Palpation is made easier with the patient in side lying with the knees drawn up to flex the hip to 90°. The whole joint line should be palpated to find the most tender area which should then be needled (Fig. 9.8).

Chest and thorax

The unique feature of the vertebrae in the thoracic region is the presence of small facets which articulate with the ribs. They form the

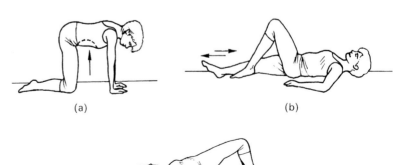

Figure 9.7. *Lumbar stabilisation exercise. Stage 1 (**a**) Abdominal hollowing, draw the abdominal muscles in a hold. (**b**) Hold the abdominal muscles tight and the pelvis still whilst moving the leg. (**c**) Bridging*

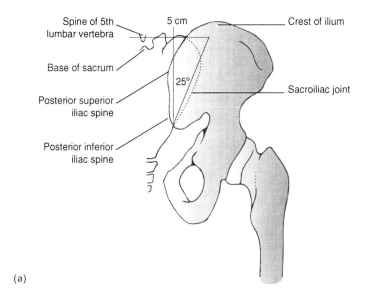

(a)

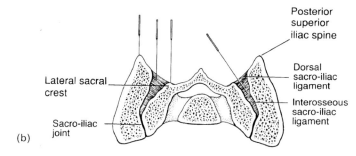

(b)

Figure 9.8. *Needling the sacro-iliac joint. (a) Surface marking. (b) Position of needles (transverse section)*

costo-vertebral joints (rib to vertebral body) and *costo-transverse* joints (rib to transverse process). The joints have loose capsules strengthened by ligaments, and may be injured through sudden twists or coughing actions. Pain is experienced to thoracic rotation and also deep/forced breathing. The rib articulates at the front with the sternum forming the *sterno-costal* joints, and also with the costal cartilages of the other ribs to form the *costo-chondral* joints.

The ribs obviously move during breathing and pivot about the various costal joints. Injury to any of these joints will affect rib movements and similarly rib injury (seat belt stress following a car accident, for example) may give pain focussed over one of the costal joints. The presence of the ribs restricts movement in the thoracic spine, particularly that of lateral flexion and flexion. Extension movements are important as they flatten the back of the rib cage providing a smooth surface for movements of the scapula during arm reaching overhead. Following injury it is the extension movement which is normally reduced and restoration of this often gives marked pain reduction.

Acupuncture treatment for the thoracic spine and ribs focusses on local points on the inner and outer bladder meridians and distal points

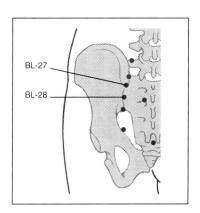

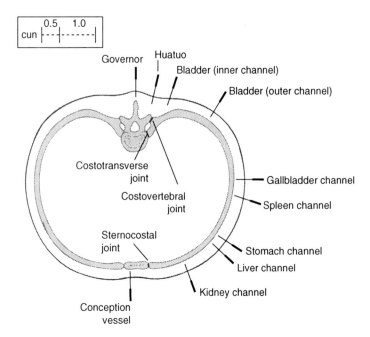

Figure 9.9. *Acupuncture points of the thorax*

including BL-60 to target pain in the whole meridian. When needling the thorax the position of the pleura and major organs must be considered. Oblique insertion *towards the spine* to a maximum depth of 0.5–1.0 cun is all that is required. Perpendicular needling, or deep oblique needling away from the spine (i.e. away from the bulk of the spinal extensor muscles and towards the ribs) carries the risk of pneumothorax. The Governor vessel points overlie the interspinous ligament and the inner bladder line points, lying 1.5 cun lateral to the lower border of the spinous processes, are close to the costo-transverse joints. The Huatuo (extra) points which are 0.5 cun lateral to the depressions below the spinous processes overlie the costo-vertebral joints. All may be palpated at the level of the lesion and needled if painful.

The sterno-costal joints must again be needled with caution, noting the potential for puncturing the lung. The kidney channel lies 0.5 cun from the midline up to KI-21 at the level of the sterno-costal angle, and then moves out to 2.0 cun from the midline in the 5th intercostal space (KI-22). It remains at this distance to its terminal point at KI-27 in the depression below the lower border of the medial clavicle. The Conception points lie directly on the midline. Transverse or transverse oblique needling is used directing the needle laterally along the intercostal space for the kidney channel, and superiorly or inferiorly along the sternum for the Conception vessel points. The maximum depth even for transverse oblique needling is 0.5 cun. The needle remains in the skin and must not penetrate further. Acupuncture aimed at needling into the intercostal muscles is fraught with danger. Manual therapy alone should be used.

The stomach channel lies 4.0 cun from the midline (on the mamillary or 'nipple' line) from ST-18 in the 5th intercostal space up to ST-12 above the midpoint of the clavicle. The liver channel affects the lower

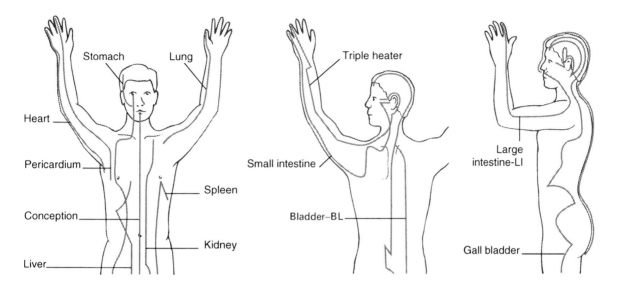

Figure 9.10. *Channels crossing the thorax*

ribs with LR-13 lying at the free end of the 11th rib and LR-14 positioned 4.0 cun from the midline in the 6th intercostal space. The gallbladder channel lies in relation to the liver channel over the lower ribs with GB-26 positioned directly below LR-13 and GB-24 below LR-14. The channel then moves to the mid axillary line, GB-22 lying in the 5th intercostal space. The spleen channel lies 4.0 cun from the midline up to SP-16, 3 cun above the umbilicus where it then moves out to a line 6.0 cun from the midline, SP-17 lying in the 5th intercostal space. The channel continues on this line to SP-20 in the 2nd intercostal space where it then turns back on itself to terminate at SP-21 in the mid axillary line in the 6th intercostal space (see also Fig. 7.14, page 130). Although too distant from the sterno-costal joints, stomach, liver, gallbladder and spleen points may be of use in the treatment of rib or intercostal muscle pain. Again cautious needling is required. A transverse oblique insertion is used along the intercostal space to a maximum depth of 0.5 cun.

Manual therapy to the thoracic spine typically uses extension and rotation mobilisations to restore pain-free movements to the spine. For extension mobilisation (postero-anterior vertebral pressure) palpation is made either with the practitioner's thumbs or the pisiform bone at the side of the hand. Gentle, rhythmical oscillation is used to restore pain free movement (Fig. 9.11a). Rotation mobilisation is carried out in sitting with the practitioner standing behind the patient (Fig. 9.11b). Pressure is imposed over the transverse processes of the thoracic vertebrae with the practitioner's hypothenar eminence at the ulnar side of the hand.

Manual therapy for the sterno-costal joints is performed by palpating the rib at the required level and performing an oscillatory mobilisation. The gaps between the ribs should be assessed and compared by palpation. Where restricted movement is detected the rib below the stiff

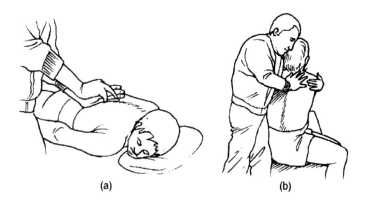

Figure 9.11. *Manual therapy of the thoracic spine*

(a)   (b)

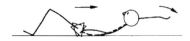

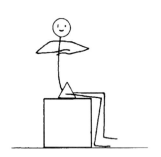

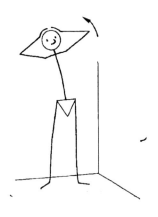

Figure 9.12. *Exercise therapy of the thorax.*

segment is gripped with the practitioner's finger tips and the patient instructed to take a deep breath and hold it for 5–10 seconds. In this way any scar tissue in the intercostal muscles resulting from direct trauma or rib fracture, for example, may be stretched out. Local massage to the intercostal muscles is also of benefit.

Exercise therapy targets extension, rotation, and lateral flexion movements of the thoracic spine (Fig. 9.12). In each case it is important to ensure that the movement is occurring at the thoracic spine and not the lumbar spine instead. The abdominal muscles should be tightened and held tight throughout the exercise to stabilise (fixate) the lumbar spine and make the thoracic spine move instead.

Cervical spine

The cervical spine consists of seven vertebra categorised into two functional units. The sub-occipital region (below the head) comprises the occiput of the skull and the first and second cervical vertebrae (C1 and C2). The lower cervical region comprises the second cervical vertebra through to the first thoracic vertebra (C2 to T1). One of the common and important postural abnormalities in the cervical spine is the forward head posture. In this posture the chin pokes forward, normally as a result of prolonged computer screen usage or deskwork. In this position, the lower cervical region is flexed and tends to stiffen in this position. This alignment causes the patient to look downward, and obviously they would not be able to walk normally like this, so to compensate they hyperextend the sub-occipital region of the cervical spine. This in turn places stress on the posterior structures by 'squashing' the facet joints. In all cases of cervical pain therefore it is important to assess movement of the sub-occipital region relative to that of the lower cervical area. Restoration of correct alignment should be a secondary aim following all acupuncture treatments of prolonged cervical pain.

An important feature of the cervical spine is the presence of the vertebral arteries. These begin as branches from the subclavian artery and run through the transverse foramen of each cervical vertebra from C6 upwards. They supply 11 per cent of the total cerebral blood flow (the carotid arteries supplying the rest) and can be a cause of headaches if compressed. Importantly injury to the vertebral arteries can be life-threatening making manipulation of the cervical spine a highly specialised form of treatment.

For acupuncture treatment of the sub-occipital region two points are of particular use, GV-16 in the depression below the external occipital protuberance and GB-20, midway between this point and the mastoid process. GB-20 (wind pool) is a major point to eliminate wind, and as such very useful in the treatment of neck pain made worse by wind and cold, and that involving headache. Similarly GV-16 (palace of wind) also eliminates winds and treats sub-occipital headache. BL-10 may also be selected if painful. Suitable distal points include GB-39 (influential point for marrow) or GB-40 (source point). Periosteal needling along the attachment of the trapezius muscle to the nuchal line is also beneficial if this area is tender to palpation (Fig. 7.2, page 126).

For the lower cervical area GV-14, below the spine of the 7th cervical vertebra (C7) is of benefit where there is an underlying deficiency such as arthritis. This point is the meeting point of the six yang channels and is particularly adept at clearing pathogens from these channels and 'firming the exterior' of the body. Inner bladder channel points may be used if painful and BL-11, level with the 1st thoracic vertebra (T1) may be chosen for its additional function as the influential point for bones. Increased muscle tension and active trigger points may be detected in the upper trapezius (GB-21), supraspinatus (TE-15 or SI-12) and infraspinatus (SI-11) and these points serve as the starting point for palpation seeking positive jump signs.

A number of distal points may be used in cases of cervical pain (Maciocia, 1994). SI-3 may be used for pain over the occiput and back of the neck along the bladder channel. This point treats the Major Yang (Tai-yang) channels (small intestine and bladder). TE-5 may be used when the pain is on the side of the neck as this point belongs to the Minor Yang (Shao-yang) channels (Triple Energiser and gallbladder). GB-39 (see above) is useful where movement range is limited and BL-60 in cases of chronic pain.

For acute neck pain such as torticollis, an extra point *Luozhen* may be of use. This is similar in effect to that of ST-38 with acute shoulder pain. The point is needled to a depth of 0.5–1.0 cun as the patient attempts to move their neck. As with ST-38 however, this point is only really effective clinically with acute pain and movement limitation through muscle spasm. Luozhen is located on the dorsum of the hand between the 2nd and 3rd MCP joints. The point lies in a small depression just proximal to the joints and is needled with the hand resting in a loose fist. In this position the prominences of the MCP joints and Luozhen form a triangle.

Torticollis may also be treated with local points close to the sternomastoid muscle. LI-18 and ST-9 lie posterior and anterior to the sternomastoid muscle bellies at the level of the laryngeal prominence (Adam's apple). GB-12 may be used in addition as it lies close to the mastoid process, part of the insertion of the sternomastoid muscle.

Manual therapy and exercise therapy are an important addition to acupuncture treatment. Manual traction of the cervical spine is helpful with a slow continuous pressure being used. Rotation mobilisations are also helpful, usually performed away from the painful side. The practitioner grasps the patient's chin and occiput and uses a gentle

Clinical note

Palpation of the cervical spine and skull base

With the patient in prone lying several structures may be palpated. Just below the centre of the posterior portion of the skull (occipital bone) lies the external occipital protuberance (EOP) and extending laterally from this the nuchal lines. Approximately 5 cm above the EOP the three major sutures of the skull meet, creating the posterior fontanelle in the child and the Lambda in the adult. Moving the palpating fingers laterally, just behind the ear the mastoid processes may be felt. Moving down from the EOP the external occipital crest can be felt and beneath it a hollow level with the tubercle of the atlas bone (C1). Approximately 3 cm below the EOP lies the spine of the axis bone (C2) and close under this the spine of C3. Lower down the spinous processes of C6, C7 and T1 can be felt. Palpating the upper two 'bumps' (C6 and C7) ask the patient to lift their head. With cervical extension the spinous process of C6 moves forwards and that of C7 stays put. To confirm the level, ask the patient to prop themselves up onto their elbows and rotate their neck while palpating the two lower 'bumps'. C7 will move with cervical rotation and T1 will not.

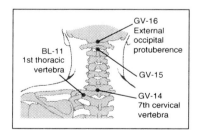

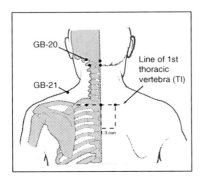

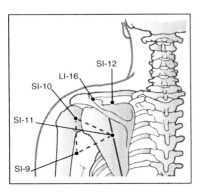

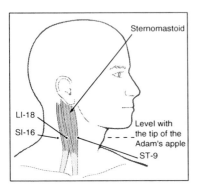

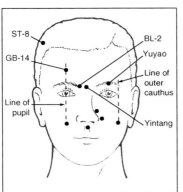

oscillation to encourage rather than force movement. Correction of a head forward cervical posture (if present) is essential. The patient should stand with their back against a wall. The action is to slowly draw (tuck) the chin in without looking downwards or upwards, in an attempt to touch the wall with the back of the skull. Five to 10 repetitions should be performed, gradually increasing the movement range.

Headache

Headache is a common symptom associated with neck pain either through prolonged postural stress or trauma (whiplash). Headache and neck pain usually occur at the same time and may be frontal, occipital or temporal in nature. Importantly headaches of cervical origin do not normally change sides. Pain is aching or boring in nature and is usually of moderate intensity but not excruciating. Several associated symptoms exist including nausea, blurring of vision, dizziness and light-headedness. Pain may be continuous or episodic, and neck pain is usually a precipitating factor. Sustained neck postures are a common provoking factor. Upper cervical extension with a forward head posture is common, and is often associated with thickening in the sub-occipital tissues.

From a TCM point of view, there are three headache patterns. The first is due to the invasion of pathogenic *wind* into the upper meridians crossing the head. Secondly excessive yang in the *liver* causing it to rise upwards, and thirdly headache due to *deficiency* of qi and blood.

Headache due to pathogenic invasion by wind is made worse by exposure to this pathogen. The pain is intense and often extends down to the neck and upper back. Upsurge of liver yang presents as irritability, a flushed face and a rapid pulse. There is often blurring of vision (liver opens to the eye) and the eyelid may be affected. There may be bilateral pain at the side of the head due to the effect on the gallbladder meridian (internally/externally linked to the liver channel). Liver headaches are made worse by heat and the patient often likes to be in a cold room or to place their head on a cool pillow. Headache due to deficiency is often associated with tiredness. This type of headache is eased by warmth and made worse by cold. Overwork may bring the headache on as it consumes further qi. The area of headache indicates the channel affected (Table 9.2).

Table 9.2. Headache locations.

Location	Channel indicated	Points recommended
Occipital (back of head) and sub-occipital (nape of neck)	Bladder	GB-20, BL-60, SI-3
Frontal (forehead) and supraorbital (above eye)	Stomach	ST-8, Yintang (extra), GV-23, LI-4, ST-44
Temporal (side of head)	Gallbladder (secondary to liver)	Taiyang (extra) GB-8, TE-5, GB-41
Parietal (top or 'cap' of head)	Liver	GV-20, SI-3, BL-67, LR-3

(Xinnong, 1999)

Where headache is due to pathogenic invasion of wind, the aim of acupuncture treatment is to remove the obstruction and dispel the wind. A reducing method is used. For occipital pain gallbladder and bladder points are chosen. GB-20 is a major point due to its ability to eliminate wind. BL-60 may be used as a distal point to 'pacify wind' and alleviate pain. Frontal pain targets the stomach meridian with ST-8 at the corner of the hairline being the local point and ST-44 (heavenly star point) the distal. Yintang (extra) at the midpoint of the eyebrows may also be used. Temporal headaches use GB-8 above the apex of the ear as a local point and GB-40 or GB-41 as a distal point. TE-5 is an important point for any headache but especially temporal headaches and those due to the liver. The extra point Taiyang, posterior to the corner of the eye, may also be used. Parietal headaches are treated with GV-20 (top of the head) as a local point and LR-3 as a distal point. SI-3 may be used to benefit the occiput and to regulate the Governing vessel. LI-4 may be used for any disorder of the head, face, or sense organs.

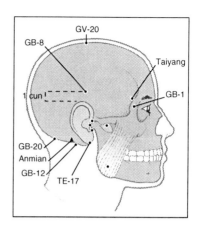

For deficiency headache a reinforcing technique is used and ST-36 may be added for its effect of producing more qi and blood. Traditionally, back shu points of the kidney (BL-23), spleen (BL-20) and liver (BL-18) would also be used. Liver headaches target LR-2 and GB-43. The former as the sedation point of the liver meridian and the latter as a 'spring point' indicated for 'heat in the body'.

Where either headache or neck pain is associated with insomnia, the extra point Anmian ('peaceful sleep') may be used. This point is located midway between GB-20 and TE-17 (see page 100).

Temporo-mandibular joint

Pain from the temporo-mandibular joint (TMJ) can refer pain into the face and head and must be distinguished from that of cervical origin. The joint is positioned between the mandibular fossa of the temporal bone and the condyle of the mandible. The joint is controlled by three main muscles, the temporalis, masseter and pterigoids. Acupuncture treatment targeted at the temporalis and masseter muscles in particular can be effective. At rest the upper teeth usually lie in front of the lower ones. As the mouth is opened the lower teeth move down and forward, causing gliding and rotation movements at the TMJ. The masseter muscles close the mouth powerfully and can develop trigger points in cases of teeth grinding. The lateral pterigoid pulls the mandible forward (protraction) and the temporalis pulls it back (retraction). Patients with TMJ pathology often present with a dull ache over the side of the face and may have limited opening of the mouth.

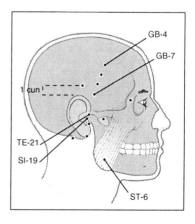

Acupuncture treatment targets local points of the joint and trigger points of the muscles. Either SI-19 ('palace of hearing') or TE-21 ('ear gate') may be chosen as the local points related to the joint. ST-6 is used as the local point in the centre of the masseter muscle. Palpation along the gallbladder line from in front of the upper ear (GB-7) to the corner of the hairline (GB-4) may elicit a trigger point in the temporalis muscle which should be needled.

Manual therapy includes distraction, with the practitioner pressing down on the lower jaw to encourage greater opening. Medial and lateral gliding is facilitated by the practitioner holding over the chin with the web of the hand and stabilising the head with the opposite hand.

Upper limb treatment protocols

Shoulder

The shoulder is an area where pain can cause marked limitation of movement and so acupuncture can have dramatic results. The back of the shoulder and scapular region is covered by the small intestine meridian while the outer aspect of the arm and top of the shoulder is covered by the large intestine and Triple Energiser meridians. These yang channels are coupled to the yin channels on the anterior aspect of the arm, the lung, heart, and pericardium.

Pain to abduction

When pain limits range of motion in the shoulder, two types of injury are common. Impingement pain occurs when a structure, usually the supraspinatus muscle or the long head of the biceps muscle, becomes trapped within the sub-acromial arch. This is the area formed below the coracoacromial ligament which provides a link between the corocoid process and the acromion process of the scapula. Capsular limitation occurs when the joint capsule tightens as a result of joint inflammation. Limitation is in a set pattern, with abduction and lateral rotation of the gleno-humeral joint being particularly limited and medial rotation being slightly limited. Where the capsule alone is affected, flexion and adduction are generally less affected than the other movements described.

Where impingement is the source of pain and movement limitation, abduction to 90° followed by medial rotation squeezes the trapped structure and reproduces the patient's pain (Hawkins's sign). Where capsular limitation is present, overhead reaching actions which combine abduction with lateral rotation often cause pain. The pain with impingement is a sudden 'pinching' feeling which occurs as the arm approaches the horizontal position and may reduce or disappear as the arm is taken overhead, a so-called 'painful arc' of movement. The

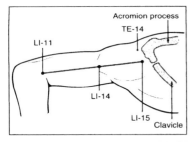

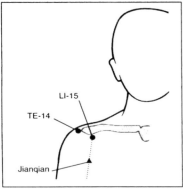

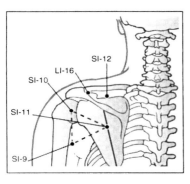

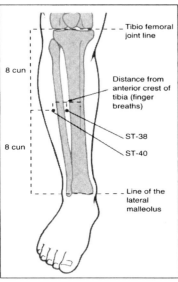

pain from capsular stretch occurs at the end of the range of motion (there is no painful arc) and comes on, gradually increasing as the arm is stretched still further.

Several acupuncture points are classically used for shoulder pain. LI-15 and TE-14 are described as the 'eyes of the shoulder' lying anterior and posterior to the acromion process. Where the pain is focussed on the anterior aspect of the joint the extra point *Jianqian* should be palpated and needled if tender. These points may be combined with LI-11 (heavenly star point). This point is especially important in cases of painful obstruction syndrome where wind is a pathogen (wandering bi). Where the pain is on the top of the shoulder directly over the supraspinatus muscle (not the tendon) LI-16 is used. For pain focussed on the posterior aspect of the shoulder small intestine points are used, either SI-9 or SI-10 being chosen. Both points alleviate pain in the posterior aspect of the shoulder, but SI-9 has a greater effect on wind as a pathogen whereas SI-10 is closer to the joint and is the meeting point for the three major meridians; crossing the back of the shoulder, the small intestine meridian, yang linking and yang motility vessels. Using a combination of SI-10, TE-14, LI-15 and Jianqian will completely surround the gleno-humeral joint. Where there is lateral pain radiating from the shoulder towards the elbow, LI-14 may be used in addition to LI-15 and LI-11. In all cases of shoulder pain LI-4 may be used as the source point of the large intestine channel. However it is particularly effective if the shoulder pain is part of a general picture which involves facial pain as a component.

Where large intestine points are used, in principle the lung may also be supported by needling LU-7 (luo-connecting point) or LU-9 (source point). However caution should be used because the lung is an organ particularly susceptible to external pathogens. Generally lung points should only be used in cases of shoulder pain if there are related symptoms of this organ (see page 15).

In cases of acute shoulder pain with severely limited range of motion, ST-38 should be used on the same side as the pain. Once deqi has been obtained the patient should try to move the shoulder as the practitioner continues to manipulate the needle. Range of motion is sometimes dramatically increased in very acute cases, and local points are then needled to continue the treatment

Physical therapy techniques are used in parallel with acupuncture, and include joint mobilisation procedures and exercise for stability, muscle strength, and flexibility. Longitudinal mobilisation to disengage the gleno-humeral joint is useful. The patient should be encouraged to relax and the practitioner gently tries to ease the head of the humerus away from the glenoid with rhythmical traction oscillations. Passively moving the head of the humerus backwards and forwards in the glenoid (postero-anterior gleno-humeral joint movement) is also of value. For this procedure the arm may be by the patient's side initially and then taken into greater ranges of abduction as pain permits (Fig. 10.1). Where pain occurs at 90° abduction, inferior gliding in abduction is effective. The patient lies supine and the practitioner stands by his/her side gripping the upper arm and placing the web of the hand over the upper portion of the humerus. The action is to press the humerus downwards without allowing any side flexion of the body. The movement may also be practised in sitting, and the practitioner may use his/her knee close to the patient's ribs to prevent any

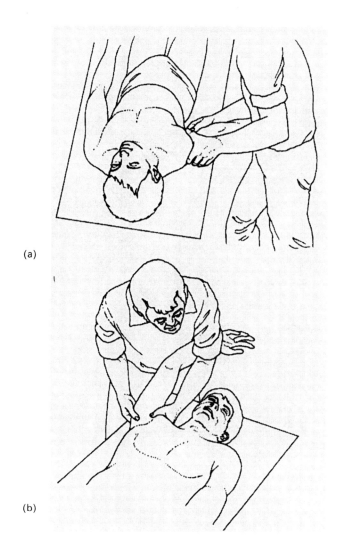

(a)

(b)

Figure 10.1. *Postero-anterior gleno-humeral joint movement. (a) 45° extension. (b) Maximal flexion-abduction*

unwanted upper body movement (Fig. 10.2). A final stretch may be used with the patient's relaxed arm overhead. This would only be used where acupuncture has relieved pain and the final range of motion is limited. The practitioner stands at the end of the couch and places his/her knee on the couch. The patient's semi-flexed arm is taken overhead in rhythmic oscillations each of which is blocked by the practitioner's knee. By moving his/her knee away from the patient's shoulder gradually, the practitioner can increase the range of motion in a controlled, progressive fashion (Fig. 10.3).

Exercise therapy must take into account the biomechanics of shoulder movement (see Norris, 1998), known as 'gleno-humeral rhythm'. Before movement can be successful in the shoulder, stability of the scapula (shoulder blade) on the rib cage must be regained. This involves teaching the patient to draw (pull) their scapulae 'down and inward' and to hold this position for gradually increasing periods of time, up to 30–60 seconds. Once this has been achieved exercises for the shoulder joint proper may be begun, but with each exercise the shoulder

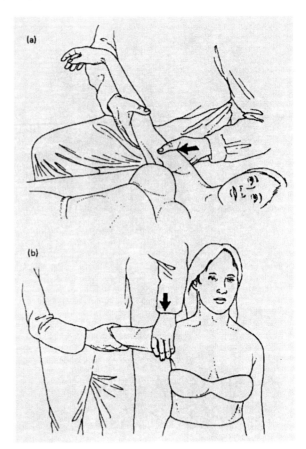

Figure 10.2. *Inferior gliding of the gleno-humeral joint. (**a**) Supine and (**b**) sitting position*

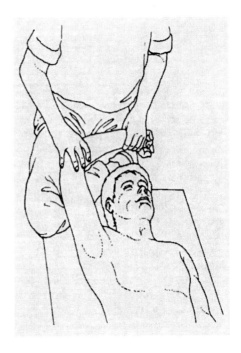

Figure 10.3. *Gleno-humeral mobilisations with the arm overhead*

alignment should be noted. The patient should be encouraged to hold the scapula firm against the ribcage rather than allowing the shoulder to shrug or the scapula to move away from the ribcage and stick out ('wing') in an obvious fashion.

Pendular swinging actions are useful for the patient to practice at home to maintain the additional movement gained during treatment. For these actions the patient should bend over from the hips and place the uninjured arm on a table. The other arm hangs down, its weight gradually pulling the humerus away from the glenoid. The action is a gentle circular swinging movement keeping the arm straight and moving from the shoulder alone. Little effort should be put into this with body movement providing some of the momentum to allow the shoulder muscles to relax.

The 'ball' (head of the humerus) of the shoulder is considerable larger than the 'socket' (glenoid) and so to keep the two together the joint capsule and ligaments are assisted by the rotator cuff muscles which lie deep to the deltoid. These muscles must always be redeveloped following shoulder injury. Resisted medial and lateral rotation are both performed with the elbow bent to 90°. Lateral rotation is especially important as it is this movement which allows the moving humerus to clear the arch at the top of the scapula as the arm is taken up towards the horizontal. Combinations of abduction and lateral rotation (thumb pointing towards the ceiling) are also used.

Stretching exercises aim to increase the available range of motion at the gleno-humeral joint and to stretch out the limited lateral rotation that is often present with tightness in the joint capsule. Two home exercises are of particular benefit (Fig. 10.4). In the first the patient kneels on all fours and grips with his/her hands onto the edge of a mat. They then sit back onto their ankles leaving their hands where they are. This has the effect of tractioning the joint and stretching it forward and overhead (flexion-abduction). The second exercise stretches rotation. The unaffected arm is placed in the small of the back and the affected (painful) arm reaches overhead and is placed between the shoulder blades. The patient attempts to join his/her hand together, initially through a towel and eventually without the towel. The exercise is then reversed.

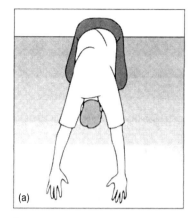

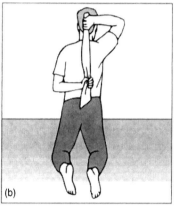

Figure 10.4. *Shoulder stretching.* **(a)** *Overhead and* **(b)** *rotation*

Tendonitis

The four most common muscles to develop tendonitis around the shoulder are the supraspinatus, infraspinatus, and subscapularis (rotator cuff) together with the long head of biceps. All may be injured through a sudden jerking action or through overuse. Tendonitis, if long standing, may develop into capsular limitation, or may present as impingement, so the treatment described above has relevance to these conditions as well. However, the individual tendons themselves may also be targeted with both local and periosteal acupuncture points.

A differential diagnosis is required to accurately distinguish the affected tissue. The supraspinatus will give pain to resisted lateral rotation and abduction. The infraspinatus gives pain to resisted lateral rotation but not to abduction. The subscapularis gives pain to resisted medial rotation of the shoulder. The long head of biceps gives pain not

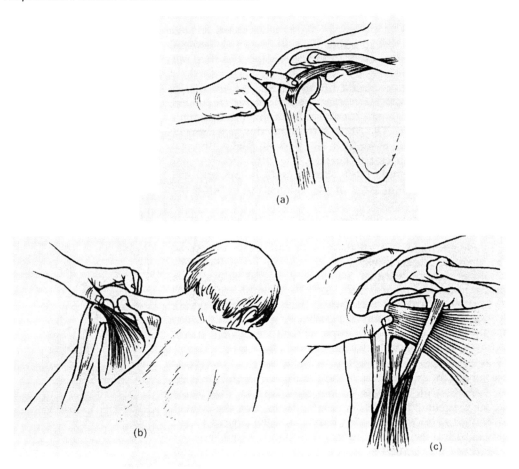

Figure 10.5. *Palpation and deep massage of the rotator cuff tendons. (a) Supraspinatus tendon. (b) Infraspinatus. (c) Subscapularis*

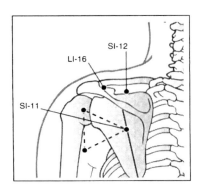

to shoulder movements alone, but to resisted elbow flexion and supination. The location of the pain is also important. Medial rotation (hand in the small of the back) brings the supraspinatus tendon to the fore by stretching it over the greater tuberosity of the humerus. It may be palpated approximately 1 cun below the anterior tip of the acromion. The subscapularis and the long head of biceps may be palpated in the bicipital groove of the humerus. The infraspinatus is palpated (with the patient in prone lying propped up on their elbows) over the posterior aspect of the greater tuberosity with the humerus flexed, adducted and laterally rotated.

Each of these points may be tender to palpation and effectively used as an ahshi point. In addition, SI-11 may be used to target the bulk of infraspinatus and SI-12 that of supraspinatus. LI-16 may be used for the musculotendinous junction of supraspinatus. Periosteal needling of the corocoid may be used to target the short head of biceps and also the pectoralis minor, a muscle which is commonly tight in 'round shouldered' postures. Extreme care and accurate palpation is needed when using this area due to the proximity to the pleura. In each case the traditional point provides the practitioner with the site to begin his/her search for tender areas, the tender area itself being needled.

Several trigger points are commonly found around the shoulder and may refer pain into the neck and/or arm. The superficial nature of the

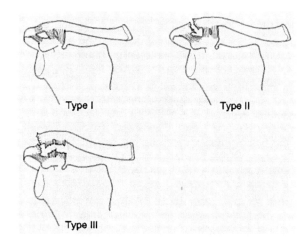

Type I   Type II

Type III

Figure 10.6. *Acromioclavicular joint injuries. Type I (sprain), type II (subluxation), type III (dislocation)*

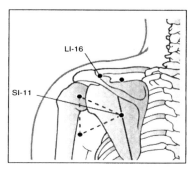

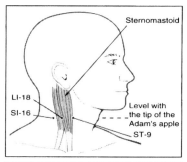

muscles makes them easy to palpate, and local pain, a taught band or a positive twitch response can usually be found. Several traditional points provide the site to begin the search for active trigger points. GB-20 for sternomastoid and the upper trapezius, GB-21 for the middle fibres of trapezius, SI-11 for the infraspinatus, the outer bladder line (BL-12/13/14) for the rhomboids, SI-16 and LI-18 for the sternomastoid, and SI-14 for the levator scapulae.

Exercise is vital in parallel with acupuncture for the treatment of tendonitis of the shoulder. Resisted exercise and stretching exercise for both the medial and lateral rotators (whichever is being treated) as detailed above, will continue the benefits of the acupuncture treatment session.

In addition, deep massage techniques may also be used over the affected muscle tendon. For this technique the tendon is placed on stretch by adopting a specific body position (Fig. 10.5). The massage technique uses a transverse movement across the breadth of the tendon. Pressure is required for the skin and palpating finger to move as a single unit. If the finger simply moves across the skin, an abrasion will result and the skin is receiving the treatment effect rather than the tendon.

Sternoclavicular/Acromioclavicular joints

The sternoclavicular (S/C) and acromioclavicular (A/C) joints are typically injured through trauma either directly to the clavicle through a blow, or from a fall onto the outstretched hand. A/C dislocation (sprung shoulder) is common in sports such as rugby football and gives a classic 'step' deformity on the top of the shoulder. Various degrees of injury and displacement are seen depending on the amount of soft tissue damage which has occurred. Damage to the acromioclavicular ligament will occur in almost all injuries, but the coroco-acromio ligament and the coroco-clavicular ligaments will only be injured with greater amounts of force. Where these ligaments have been injured the clavicle will displace further and a greater step deformity is produced. The injury progresses from a simple sprain to subluxation and finally full dislocation (Fig. 10.6). The S/C joint is rarely injured, the clavicle fracturing or the A/C joint dislocating first. However, following a

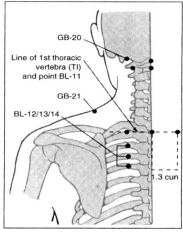

Clinical note

Joint palpation

The A/C joint lies at the lateral end of the clavicle approximately 2 cms medial to the lateral border of the acromion. The end of the clavicle is slightly raised as it borders onto the A/C joint and the joint line lies just lateral to this point. It is more easily palpated by running a finger along the superior aspect of the lateral clavicle until it reaches this raised point. The S/C joint is palpated at the medial end of the clavicle, at the upper lateral corner of the manubrium of the sternum. The joint line is curved (concave laterally) and about 1 cm long, the lower portion articulating with the clavicle, the upper portion standing slightly proud of the clavicle when the joint is not moving. The lower portion of the joint borders onto the costal cartilage of the 1st rib.

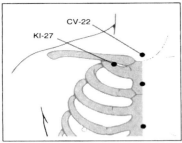

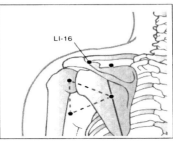

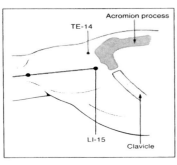

heavy lateral force imposed on the shoulder, (falling from a horse), the joint may be involved. If the clavicle is forced backwards it may impinge on the trachea, a life-threatening injury. Fortunately anterior dislocation is more common and the joint may spontaneously relocate with an audible thud as the arm is moved.

A number of traditional acupuncture points exist in relation to these joints including KI-27 and CV-22 for the S/C joint and LI-15, LI-16 and TE-14 for the A/C joint. However, periosteal needling probably provides the best route to successful treatment. The joints are palpated and tender areas needled. In each case the needle may be placed at the most painful point along the joint line.

With an acute A/C joint dislocation, taping may be used following acupuncture, to take some of the weight off the joint. A felt pad is placed over the lateral aspect of the clavicle and elastic taping passed over the shoulder to adhere to anchors placed around the chest. An anchor may also be placed on the arm and strips taken up from the upper arm over the top of the shoulder to the middle of the clavicle. These will have the effect of taking some of the weight of the arm and reducing the traction force on the joint (Fig. 10.7).

Joint mobilisation techniques are an essential complement to acupuncture treatment, and focus on moving the clavicle relative to the sternum or scapula. Minimal gliding movements are used, either pressing on the anterior aspect of the clavicle or pressing from above, in each case with the patient lying supine. With the patient sitting, postero-anterior movements are also possible. The practitioner presses the clavicle from behind.

Elbow

Elbow injuries all tend to be popularly grouped under the term 'tennis elbow' although in reality it is only a lesion to the common extensor origin over the lateral epicondyle which is covered by this term. Pain over the medial epicondyle (common flexor origin) should be described as 'golfer's elbow'.

Tennis elbow may occur to one of four sites around the common extensor origin. The most common site is the attachment of the extensor carpi radialis brevis muscle on to the epicondyle (an area called the teno-periosteal junction), but the extensor carpi radialis longus may also be affected rising up on to the supracondylar ridge of the humerus. The extensor muscles themselves may be pulled at the area of tissue that forms a bridge between the tendon and muscle – the musculotendinous junction. Both traditional and western acupuncture approaches have merit in the treatment of this condition.

Points along the large intestine meridian are selected for tennis elbow. LI-11 being a local point with LI-10 added for pain within the muscle belly. Occasionally LI-12 (I cun above LI-11) may be chosen for pain, spreading up onto the supracondylar ridge. LI-4 (source point) is used as a distal point. LU-5 may also be used partly as a local point and partly because the lung meridian is internally/externally linked to the large intestine meridian. Periosteal points are often located at the lateral epicondyle itself and are painful to needle, but the

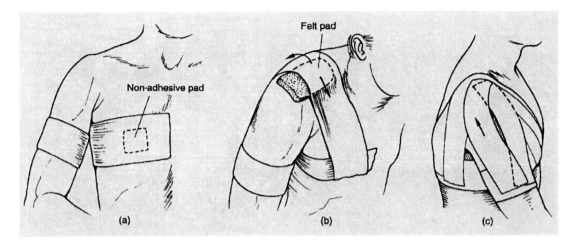

results are largely very good. The most tender point is palpated and the needle inserted. A 'pecking' or 'peppering' technique is used covering an area about 0.5 cm in diameter.

In some cases inflammation may have spread from the lateral epicondyle to the head of the radius, and in these cases periosteal needling to the radial head may be tried. This technique is also of use following a reduced radial head dislocation (swinging small children by the arms). The head of the radius lies just below the lateral epicondyle of the humerus. If both points are palpated, the radial head will obviously move with pronation and supination, the epicondyle will not. The joint space itself lies beneath the anconeus muscle and so cannot be accurately palpated.

Golfer's elbow gives medial pain, and the muscles involved are the pronator teres and the flexor carpi radialis attaching to the medial epicondyle. For this condition the small intestine meridian is used. SI-8, lying at the elbow between the tip of the medial epicondyle and the olecranon process of the ulna may be used with SI-4 (source point) or SI-3 (confluence point, to bring in the yang motility vessel) as a distal point. HT-3 may also be used as a local point. Again, periosteal needling is of particular importance if pain spreads up onto the epicondyle itself.

Trigger points may be found in the extensor carpi radialis longus or brevis and occasionally in the supinator or extensor digitorum (tennis elbow), and in the pronator teres and flexor carpi radialis (golfer's elbow). These muscles should be palpated firstly with the elbow pronated and then with it supinated. Where a positive twitch response or reproduction of pain is found, that point should be needled.

With both tennis elbow and golfer's elbow the addition of periosteal needling and painful local (ahshi) points, rather than traditional points alone, normally gives a better result.

Exercise is a procedure often frowned on with tennis elbow as the pain is seen as an overuse injury. In reality however, correctly applied exercise therapy is a vital component of treatment as pain begins to ease with acupuncture. Two exercises are useful to restore the strength and endurance to the forearm extensor muscles. The first uses the muscles as stabilisers to 'lock' the wrist, the second uses the same muscles as prime movers, to 'activate' the wrist. Both functions are vital to full

Figure 10.7. *Acromioclavicular joint taping. (a) Anchors. (b) Stirrup applied under tension. (c) Arm stirrups*

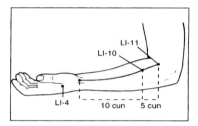

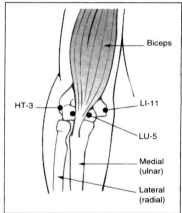

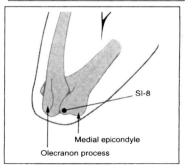

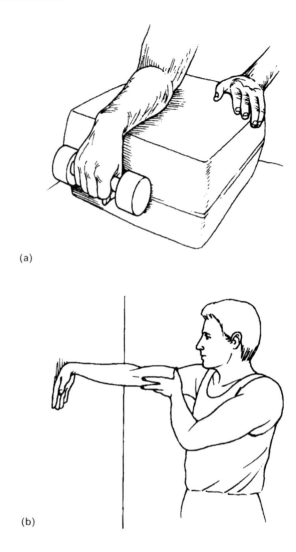

(a)

(b)

Figure 10.8. *Exercise therapy for tennis elbow.* **(a)** *Resisted forearm extension.* **(b)** *Forearm extensor stretch against a wall*

rehabilitation. The first exercise is known in sport as a 'reverse curl'. The patient grips a weight (a can of food or small dumbbell) and holds their elbow tucked into their side. With the knuckles facing the ceiling the action is to bend and straighten the elbow *without moving the wrist.* The second exercise is called a 'reverse wrist curl' (Fig. 10.8a). Again the patient holds a weight but this time they place their forearm on the edge of a table. The action is to flex and extend the wrist without raising the forearm from the table. Both exercises should be performed in a slow controlled fashion to the point at which pain begins, but no further. With time more repetitions of the exercises will be possible before pain comes on. Stretching for tennis elbow is also used and can be important with long-standing injuries. With the arm straight (elbow locked), the patient places the back of their hand onto a wall and leans forwards, pressing the wrist into further flexion (Fig. 10.8b). The point of maximum stretch is held for 30 seconds and then slowly released.

For golfer's elbow the flexor muscles are targeted although these muscles are normally strong through daily activities making specific rehabilitation exercise less important.

Posterior elbow pain

Pain at the back of the elbow is seen after a rapid hyperextension action of the joint such as throwing. Several structures may be implicated around the olecranon. The olecranon bursa is found at the bony point of the elbow lying directly over the olecranon process, and may become inflamed by falling or leaning heavily onto the point of the elbow. Another source of pain is the insertion of the triceps muscle onto the posterior aspect of the olecranon. This insertion may be torn or inflamed following throwing actions in sport. As the elbow is snapped backwards rapidly in throwing, the olecranon may also be forced into the fossa causing inflammation and eventually cortical bone damage and thickening if the stress continues.

The Triple Energiser channel is targeted with TE-10 (in the depression above the olecranon) and TE-11 (1 cun above) being the important local points. SI-8 (between the olecranon and the medial epicondyle) may also be used for postero-medial pain. Distal points include TE-4 (source point) and TE-5 (luo-connecting point and confluence point). TE-5 is more likely to give a good result where there is tenderness over the extensor muscles in addition to posterior elbow pain. Where the internally/externally linked yin meridian is to be supported, PC-3 (local point) or PC-7 (source point) may be chosen.

It is important to ensure that full extension of the elbow is obtained following posterior elbow conditions. Mobilisation and exercise therapy should therefore be aimed at enabling the patient to lock the elbow out fully. Re-strengthening the triceps muscle may also be required. A suitable exercise to achieve both of these aims is a triceps extension movement. The patient grips a light weight in their hand and kneels on a gym bench. They tuck the elbow of their affected arm into their side and straighten their arm in line with their trunk. The aim should be to obtain full locking of the elbow, and to hold the locked position for 3–5 seconds (Fig. 10.9).

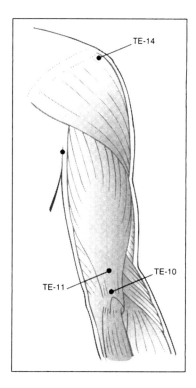

Wrist and hand

Sprain

A sprained wrist is a common 'diagnosis' but in reality only indicates the area of pain which the patient is experiencing rather than the true pathology. The tissues most commonly affected are the intercarpal ligaments, often in association with subluxation of one or more of the carpal bones. The lunate bone is the most commonly subluxed with capitate subluxation also seen, both as a result of a fall onto the outstretched hand. The wrist is held in flexion and a prominent bump is seen on the back of the hand. Reduction by manipulation is required, and acupuncture may be used to ease the pain which results from soft tissue damage.

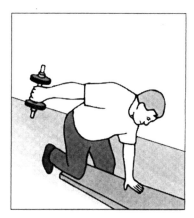

Figure 10.9. *Triceps extension exercise. Kneel on a gym bench and grip a light dumbell in the hand. Keeping the elbow tucked into the side of the body, extend the arm. Pause in the locked (straight) position and then repeat*

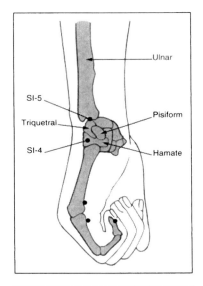

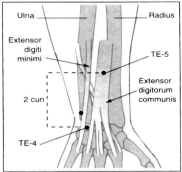

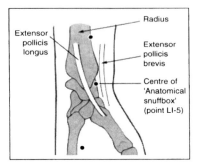

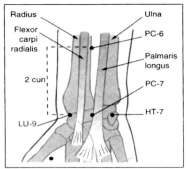

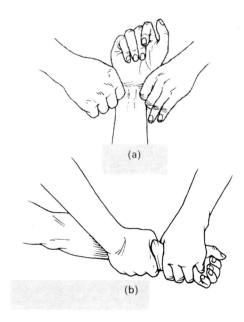

Figure 10.10. *Wrist joint mobilisation*

Acupuncture treatment targets the Triple Energiser meridian with TE-4 (source point) a focal point. TE-5 may be used as an additional local point where pain extends into the forearm. In addition, as a confluence point, TE-5 also has the effect of opening the yang linking vessel which is said to serve as an energetic template for the whole of the lateral zone (Seem, 1993). Where the wrist pain is predominantly medial (ulnar) SI-4 or SI-5 may be added, whichever is the more painful. For lateral (radial) pain LI-5 may be added.

Several mobilisation procedures are used to regain full movement at the wrist and these are used with a home exercise programme. The lower ends of the radius and ulnar may be gripped and the two bones moved relative to each other to target the inferior radioulnar joint (Fig. 10.10a). By holding the patient's hand in one hand and his/her wrist in the other, the practitioner can move the hand relative to the wrist to mobilise the radiocarpal joint (Fig. 10.10b). Wrist mobility exercises are carried out with the flat of the hand on a table top, at the edge of the table. The other hand is placed over the injured one to fix it and the forearm is moved relative to this. Flexion/extension (elbow moving up and down) and abduction/adduction (elbow moving side to side) may both be obtained.

Carpal tunnel

The carpal tunnel (Fig. 10.11) is formed by the flexor retinaculum stretching over the hollow formed between the outermost carpal bones. The flexor muscle tendons and the median nerve pass through the tunnel, and when the tendons swell (tendonitis) the nerve may be compressed. Compression can also occur if the size of the carpal tunnel is reduced through arthritic changes to the carpal bones (often

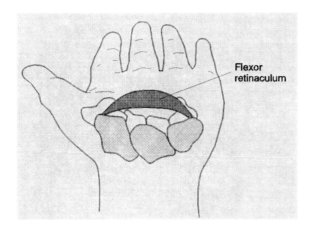

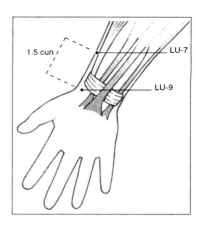

Figure 10.11. *The carpal tunnel*

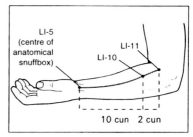

secondary to fracture) or through fluid retention. This latter cause may be seen in pregnancy or to a lesser extent during menstruation. The condition must be differentiated from pain referred from the cervical spine (C6/C7 nerve root).

The acupuncture point PC-7 is key to the effective treatment of this condition. The needle may be angled beneath the flexor retinaculum along the carpal tunnel in the direction of the hand. Both HT-7 and LU-9 may be used as additional local points lying on the flexor aspect of the wrist. PC-6 may be used as a distal point. Where the carpal tunnel syndrome exists as part of a general clinical picture involving water retention, SP-9 (systematic) or LI-11 (local) may be used to reduce the swelling. ST-36 may also be added to fortify the spleen organ's ability to resolve dampness and SP-6 used to harmonise the yin channels which are active during menstruation.

The carpal bones may be mobilised, and the flexor retinaculum stretched, by separating the pisiform, triquetral and hamate bones on one side of the wrist from the trapezium and scaphoid on the other.

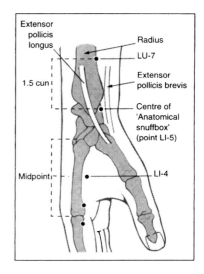

Tendonitis

Three conditions may affect the tendons at the wrist. *Tendonitis* is inflammation of the tendon itself. *Tenosynovitis* is a lesion of the gliding surfaces of the outside of the tendon and the inside of its sheath. Finally *tenovaginitis* occurs when the wall of the tendon sheath becomes chronically inflamed and actually thickens. All of the conditions can combine overuse of the tendon with compression in some way. Tendonitis to the finger tendons is seen commonly in keyboard operators. Where tenovaginitis affects the thumb (De Quervain's syndrome), it is the sheath of the abductor pollicis longus and extensor pollicis brevis tendons which is affected. The distal point of the tendon sheath can be compressed where the tendons pass over the distal aspect of the radius. There is pain and crepitus (grating) as the thumb is moved, and this is made worse when the sheath is compressed by the

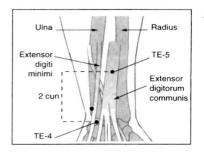

practitioner. In each case it is essential to identify the stressor likely to have precipitated the condition, and modify or remove it.

Acupuncture treatment for general posterior forearm pain targets any of the upper body yang meridians, with LI-11 and LI-4 for radial side pain, TE-9 (on a line joining the lateral epicondyle and TE-4, 7 cun proximal to the wrist crease) and TE-4 for central pain. Small intestine points may also be used for tendonitis of the flexor carpi ulnaris, although this is rare.

Where pain affects the thumb tendons, LU-9 may be used as it lies at the edge of abductor pollicus longus, one of the major muscles affected. LI-5 may also be used as a local point and LU-7 as it lies between brachioradialis and the abductor pollicis longus muscle. In addition periosteal needling of the distal aspect of the radius may also be used especially if the tendonitis is associated with arthritis of the 1st carpometacarpal (CMC) joint (see below).

Finger pain in general may be due to the finger tendons or the finger joints. Tendonitis may affect the fingers but is more usually seen over the wrist. However, tendon injury causing such conditions as Mallet finger or Trigger finger (both tendon ruptures or avulsions) are more common in sport and heavy industrial working. Pain from arthritis of the fingers or thumb is made worse by compression (the practitioner presses on the end of the patient's straight finger) and shows limitation of movement and an inability to completely lock the fingers out straight. For the CMC joint of the thumb, abduction is the movement most limited in arthritis. This is easily assessed by asking the patient to place their hands in a prayer position and spread (abduct) their thumbs. The limited range of motion becomes obvious when comparing the two hands. The collateral ligaments of the finger joints (metacarpophalangeal or interphalangeal) may be affected through trauma (a ball hitting the finger in sport). Injury to the CMC joint of the thumb is a common skiing injury, where the ulnar collateral ligament is normally injured by forced abduction.

Acupuncture treatment of finger pain includes the Baxie points, lying in the depressions between the metacarpal heads proximal to the finger webs, and for the 1st CMC joint, LU-9 and LI-5. Periosteal needling to the metacarpal heads in general is also effective (Mann, 1992). For the 1st CMC joint, periosteal needling of the carpal bones is effective. The needle is inserted to strike the scaphoid from a dorsal approach or the trapezium from either a dorsal or palmar approach, the most painful bony area being targeted. In addition the joint line of the 1st CMC joint may be chosen. This is palpable from its posterior aspect, and the practitioner's finger should slide proximally along the shaft of the 1st metacarpal to its enlarged base. Just proximal to this is a slight depression identifying the joint line which lies on either side of the tendon of extensor pollicis longus (Fig.10.12).

Stretching to the 1st CMC joint is useful, as is self traction. Stretching is carried out by gently pulling the thumb back into extension and abduction with the other hand, and holding this position for 20–30 seconds. For self traction the patient simply grips his/her thumb with the other hand and gently pulls, keeping the thumb in line. The stretch should be maintained for 5–10 seconds and repeated five times.

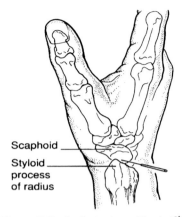

Figure 10.12. *Periosteal needling in 1st CMC pain*

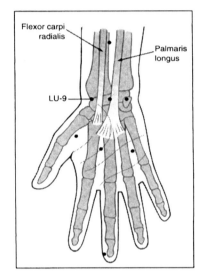

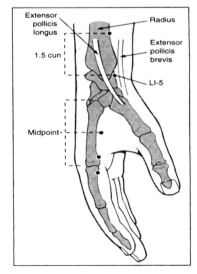

References

Awad, E.A. (1990). Histopathological changes in fibrositis. In *Advances in Pain Research and Therapy* (J.R. Fricton, and E.A. Awad, eds.) Raven Press.

Baldrey, P. (1998) Trigger point acupuncture. In *Medical Acupuncture* (J. Filshie and A. White, eds.) Churchill Livingstone.

Barlos, P. and Mak, K. (1999). *Myofascial Pain. Course Notes.* Ellesmere Port Hospital. UK.

Bowden, S.D., Davis, D.O. and Dina, T.S. (1990). Abnormal magnetic resonance scans of the lumbar spine in asymptomatic individuals. *J. Bone Joint Surg. (Am)*, **72**, 403.

Bowsher, D. (1998). Mechanisms of acupuncture. In *Medical Acupuncture* (J. Filshie and A. White, eds.) Churchill Livingstone.

Brattberg, G. (1986). Acupuncture treatments: a traffic hazard? *Am. J. Acupunct.*, **14**, 265–7.

Bray, J.J. (1986). *Lecture Notes on Human Physiology*. Blackwell Scientific Publications.

Campbell, A. (2000). *Acupuncture in Practice*. Self published. a.campbell@doctors.org.uk.

Chen, F., Hwang, S. and Lee, H. (1990). Clinical study of suncope during acupuncture treatment. *Acupunct. Electrother. Res.*, **15**, 107–19.

Chopra, D. (1998). *Healing the Heart*. Random House Audiobooks.

Corrigan, B. and Maitland G.D. (1998). *Vertebral Musculoskeletal Disorders*. Butterworth-Heinemann.

Cross, J.R. (2000). *Acupressure*. Butterworth-Heinemann.

Deadman, P., Al-Khafaji, M. and Baker, K. (1998). *A Manual of Acupuncture*. Journal of Chinese Medicine Publications.

Doutsu, Y., Tao, Y. and Sasayama, K. (1986). A case of *Staphylococcus aureus* septicemia after acupuncture therapy. *Kansenshogaku Zasshi*, **60**, 911–6.

Dundee, J.W., Ghaly, R.G., Bill, K.M., Chestnutt, W.N., Fitzpatrick, K.T.J. and Lynas, A.G.A. (1989). Effect of stimulation of the P6 antiemetic point on postoperative nausea and vomiting. *Br. J. Anaesth.*, **63**, 612–8.

Dung, H.C. (1984). Anatomical features contributing to the formation of acupuncture points. *Am. J. Acupunct.*, **12**, 139–43.

Ellis, A., Wiseman, N. and Boss, K. (1994). *Fundamentals of Chinese Acupuncture*. Revised edition. Paradigm Publications.

Field, D. (1994). *Anatomy: Palpation and Surface Markings*. Butterworth-Heinemann.

Filshie, J. and White, A. (1998). *Medical Acupuncture. A Western Scientific Approach*. Churchill Livingstone.

Fujiwara, H., Taniguchi, K., Takeuchi, J. and Ikezono, E. (1980). The influence of low frequency acupuncture on a demand pacemaker. *Chest*, **78**, 96–7.

Gilbert, J.G. (1987). Auricular complications of acupuncture. *N. Z. Med. J.*, **100**, 141–2.

Halvorsen, T.B., Anda, S.S., Naess, A.B. and Levang, O.W. (1995). Fatal cardiac tamponade after acupuncture through congenital sternal foramen. *Lancet*, **345**, 1175.

Hayhoe, S. and Pitt, E. (1987). Case reports. Complications of acupuncture. *Acupuncture in Medicine*, **4**, 15.

Headley, B.J. (1990). EMG and myofascial pain. *Clin. Management*, **10**(4), 43–6.

Heine, H. (1988). Akupunkturtherapie-Perforationen der oberflachlichen Korperfazie durch kutane Gefab-Nervenbundel. *Therapeutikon*, **4**, 238–44.

Izatt, E. and Fairman, M. (1977). Staphylococcal septicaemia with DIC associated with acupuncture. *Postgrad. Med. J.*, **53**, 285–6.

James, R. (1993). Linear skin rashes and the meridians of acupuncture. *Eur. J. Orient. Med.*, **1**(1), 42–6.

Jefferys, D.B., Smith, S., Brennand-Roper, D.A. and Curry, P.V.L. (1983). Acupuncture needles as a cause of bacterial endocarditis. *Br. Med. J.*, **287**, 326-7.

Hirsch, P.W. and Nachemson, A. (1954). New observations on mechanical behaviour of lumbar discs. *Acta Orthopaed. Scand.*, **23**, 254–83.

Kaptchuk, T.J. (1983). *Chinese Medicine. The Web That Has No Weaver*. Rider.

Kirschenbaum, A.E. and Rizzo, C. (1997). Glenohumeral pyarthrosis following acupuncture treatment. *Orthopedics*, **20**, 1184–6.

Lavignolle, B., Vitral, J.M. and Senegas, J. (1983). An approach to the functional anatomy of the sacroiliac joints in *vivo*. Anat. Clin., **5**, 169–76.

Leatt, P., Reilly, T. and Troup, J.G.D. (1986). Spinal loading during circuit weight-training and running. *Br. J. Sports Med.*, **20**(3), 119–24.

Low, R. (1987). *The Acupuncture Treatment of Musculo-skeletal Conditions*. Thorsons.

Maciocia, G. (1989). *The Foundations of Chinese Medicine*. Churchill Livingstone.

Maciocia, G. (1994). *The Practice of Chinese Medicine*. Churchill Livingstone.

Mann, F. (1992). *Reinventing Acupuncture*. Butterworth-Heinemann.

Mann, F. (1998). A new system of acupuncture. In *Medical Acupuncture* (J. Filshie and A. White, eds.) Churchill Livingstone.

McKenzie, R.A. (1981). *The Lumbar Spine. Mechanical Diagnosis and Therapy*. Spinal Publications.

Nachemson, A.L. (1992). Newest knowledge of low back pain. *Clin. Orthopaed.*, **279**, 8.

Nakamura, H., Konishiike, J., Sugamura, A. and Takeno, Y. (1986). Epidemiology of spontaneous pneumothorax in women. *Chest*, **89**, 378–82.

Ni, M. (1995). The Yellow Emperor's Classic of Medicine. A New Translation of the Neijing Suwen. Shambhala.

Norheim, A.J. and Fonnebo, V. (1996). Adverse effects are more than occasional case reports: results from questionnaires among 1135 randomly selected doctors and 197 acupuncturists. *Compliment. Ther. Med.*, **4**, 8–13.

Norris, C.M. (1995). Spinal stabilisation (I). *Physiotherapy*, **81**, 4–12.

Norris, C.M. (1998). *Sports Injuries: Diagnosis and Management*. Butterworth-Heinemann.

Norris, C.M. (1999). *The Complete Guide to Stretching*. A&C Blacks.

Norris, C.M. (2000). *Back Stability*. Human Kinetics. Champaign.

Pirog, J.E. (1996). *Meridian Style Acupuncture*. Pacific View Press.

Qiu M.-L. (1993). *Chinese Acupuncture and Moxibustion*. Churchill Livingstone.

Rampes, H. (1998). Adverse reactions to acupuncture, In *Medical Acupuncture* (J. Filshie and A. White, eds.) Churchill Livingstone.

Rampes, H. and Peuker, E. (1999). Adverse effects of acupuncture. In *Acupuncture and Scientific Appraisal* (E. Ernst and A. White, eds.) Butterworth-Heinemann.

Renshu College of Traditional Chinese Medicine (1998). *Advanced Certificate in Acupuncture. Course Notes*. RCTCM.

Ross, J. (1998). *Acupuncture Point Combinations*. Churchill Livingstone.

Roth, L.U., Maret-Meric, A., Adler, R.H. and Neuenschwander, B.E. (1997). Acupuncture points have subjective (needling sensation) and objective (serum cortisol increase) specificity. *Acupuncture in Medicine*. May.

Seem, M. (1993). *A New American Acupuncture*. Blue Poppy Press.

Slater, P.E., Ben-Ishai, P. and Leventhal, P. (1988). An acupuncture-associated outbreak of hepatitis B in Jerusalem. *Eur. J. Epidemiol.*, **4**, 322–5.

Society of Biophysical Medicine. (1985). *Basic Acupuncture Course*. University of Manchester, UK.

Stark, P. (1985). Midline sternal foramen: CT demonstration. *J. Comput. Ass. Tomogr.*, **9**, 489–90.

Stux, G. and Pomeranz, B. (1998). *Basics and Acupuncture*. 4th edition, Springer.

Wei, H., Chung-Long Huang, L. and Kong, J. (1999). The substrate and properties of meridians: a review of modern research. *Acupuncture in Medicine*, **17**(2), 134.

White, A. (1999). Neurophysiology of acupuncture analgesia. In *Acupuncture and Scientific Appraisal* (E. Ernst and A. White, eds.) Butterworth-Heinemann.

Xin, Z. and Jianping, F. (1994). *A Guide Book to the Proficiency Examination for International Acupuncture and Moxibustion Professionals*. China Medico-Pharmaceutical Science and Technology Publishing House.

Xinnong, C. (1999). Chinese Acupuncture and Moxibustion. 2nd edition, Foreign Languages Press.

Index

Lightning Source UK Ltd.
Milton Keynes UK
25 October 2009

145349UK00004B/19/P